Poststructuralism, Cit and Social Policy

The impact of poststructuralism on thinking in the social sciences and humanities over the last decade has been profound. However, to date, there has been little systematic analysis of the implications of poststructuralism for the critical analysis of social policy. *Poststructuralism, Citizenship and Social Policy* shows how poststructuralist ideas can be usefully applied in the areas of welfare, health, education and science and technology policy, making particular reference to the theme of citizenship.

With the winding back of the welfare state and the emergence of 'neo-liberalism', policy makers urgently need new tools of analysis. They need to rethink the relations between citizens and the state. The chapters examine the emergence and significance of neo-liberal rule for social policies, new forms of governance implied by the new genetics and the implications for public health, the meanings of education and citizenship in the context of economic rationalism, and the role of technologies in the constitution of the self.

All the authors are based at Murdoch University, Western Australia. **Alan Petersen** is Senior Lecturer in Sociology in the School of Social Inquiry, **Ian Barns** is a Lecturer at the Institute for Science and Technology Policy, **Janice Dudley** is a Lecturer in the School of Politics and International Studies and **Patricia Harris** is Associate Professor in Sociology and Social Policy in the School of Social Inquiry.

Poststructuralism, Citizenship and Social Policy

Alan Petersen, Ian Barns,
Janice Dudley and
Patricia Harris

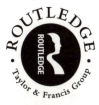

First published 1999
by Routledge
11 New Fetter Lane, London EC4P 4EE

Simultaneously published in the USA and Canada
by Routledge
29 West 35th Street, New York, NY 10001

Routledge is an imprint of the Taylor & Francis Group

© 1999 Alan Petersen, Ian Barns, Janice Dudley and Patricia Harris

Typeset in Times by The Florence Group, Stoodleigh, Devon.
Printed and bound in Great Britain by TJ International Ltd, Padstow,
Cornwall

British Library Cataloguing in Publication Data
A catalogue record for this book is available from the British Library

Library of Congress Cataloging in Publication Data
Poststructuralism, citizenship and social policy /Alan Petersen [et al.].
  p. cm.
  Includes bibliographical references and index.
  1. Social policy–Methodology. 2. Poststructuralism.
  I. Petersen, Alan R., Ph.D.
  HN28.P67 1999
  361.6'1–DC21   99–19521
                     CIP

ISBN 0–415–18287–5 (hbk)
ISBN 0–415–18288–3 (pbk)

Contents

Acknowledgements

We wish to thank Heather Gibson at Routledge, who has supported this project from the outset and who has been patient with our requests for extensions. We are grateful to Murdoch University, which has provided resources and an environment conducive to the exchange of ideas, and to the Murdoch Club, where many of our exchanges took place over coffee. Finally, we wish to thank our families and our colleagues in our respective departments at Murdoch University for their support.

Acknowledgements

Chapter 1

Introduction: themes, context and perspectives

Ian Barns, Janice Dudley, Patricia Harris and Alan Petersen

What is poststructuralism, and what has it got to do with social policy? How can policy makers, who deal with very practical issues, make use of the concepts of poststructuralism in their own work? And how does poststructural analysis relate to our understanding of citizenship? These are questions that we explore in this book, with specific reference to the social policy areas of welfare, education, public health and science and technology. In this introductory chapter, we spell out our assumptions and explain what is distinctive about our approach. We examine the politico-economic and theoretical contexts which have shaped both policy making and our own thinking, and outline the themes that are covered in the chapters that follow. We have all contributed equally to the planning and writing of this chapter. To begin, Alan explains the rationale for this book and seeks to clarify our particular use of the term 'poststructuralism', and what we believe distinguishes a poststructuralist approach from other approaches. Patricia then examines the relationship between poststructuralism and the social policy literature. This is followed by Janice's discussion of the economic and political context shaping the specific policy responses that have come to be identified with neo-liberalism. And, finally, Ian explores the relationship between citizenship and neo-liberal regimes of governance – an important recurring theme in the book – and introduces the remaining chapters.

In recent years, there has been a burgeoning number of new books focusing on poststructuralism as a theoretical perspective. There has also been a steadily growing number of texts dealing with conceptual and theoretical approaches to policy. However, as yet, few books have systematically examined the implications of poststructuralism for the critical analysis of social policy. While poststructuralism has had a profound impact on thinking in the social sciences and humanities over the last decade or so, its implications for our understandings of social policy and its impacts have been relatively unexplored. This book represents an effort to address this lacuna, to show how the insights offered by poststructuralists can be usefully employed in the analysis of contemporary social policy, with specific reference to the areas of welfare, health, education and science and technology. These are areas of our respective research interests and expertise, and also constitute much of the contemporary field of social policy. The emergence of economic liberalism, increasing globalisation, the reconstruction of the welfare state and the move towards a more market-driven approach to social provision has radically reshaped policies in all these fields, calling for new perspectives and new tools of analysis. This rapidly changing context has brought into question many of the categories and concepts by means of which we have so far understood the human, such as 'citizenship' which was developed further in the context of the welfare state. With the 'winding back' of the welfare state, the emergence of a new conservatism and attacks on established social and civil rights, it is important that policy makers and policy analysts who are concerned about protecting and advancing rights seek to critically appraise basic concepts and categories. In particular, there is a need for careful analysis of the manifestations and operations of the increasingly dominant 'rationality of rule' known as advanced liberalism or neo-liberalism. Neo-liberal policies have radically altered the public domain through privatisation, downsizing, the contracting out and rationing of services and the emphasis on local and individual autonomy. There are few areas of policy unaffected by the recent and dramatic shifts in social priorities ushered in by neo-liberal rule. In this context, the concept of citizenship is of crucial significance, as a site for exploring the meanings and limits of liberal democratic participation and for contesting the imperatives of neo-liberal rule. The concept of citizenship, with its implied rights and duties, we believe, needs to be closely and critically scrutinised at this historical juncture, and hence figures prominently in the discussion that follows.

What do we mean by poststructuralism?

Before proceeding much further, we should make clear our particular use of the term poststructuralism. Because we take seriously the claim that our descriptions are never innocent, in the sense that they are unable to provide an unmediated and impartial access to an already given social reality, but rather constitute our reality, we believe it is important that authors seek to define their terms clearly. Throughout its relatively brief history, the term poststructuralism has been charged with multiple meanings. This has led to some confusion in discussions. Confusion has arisen in part because writers often use the term 'poststructuralist' as though it were singular when in fact it is plural, encompassing diverse theoretical positions, including apparently 'apolitical' forms of deconstructive criticism and more explicit forms of political critique and practice, such as feminist poststructuralism (Weedon 1987) and queer theory (Seidman 1996). It is not our intention here to explore the diverse definitions of poststructuralism, nor the history of poststructuralist thought, since this has already been done extensively elsewhere (see, e.g., Best and Kellner 1991; Sarup 1993; Smart 1993). When we use the term poststructuralism here, we take it to mean that school of thought which is opposed to and seeks to move beyond the premises of structuralism, to develop new models of thought, writing and subjectivity. As Best and Kellner explain, structuralism focuses on the underlying rules which organise phenomena into a social system and aims at objectivity, coherence, rigour and truth. Structuralists seek to describe social phenomena in terms of linguistic and social structures, rules, codes and systems, and to develop grand, synthesising theories (Best and Kellner 1991: 19). Examples of structuralist analysis include Marxism and function-alist sociology. Poststructuralists, on the other hand, focus on the inextricable and diffuse linkages between power and knowledge, and on how individuals are constituted as subjects and given unified identities or subject positions. That is, they focus on micro politics and on subjectivity, difference and everyday life (ibid.: 24). This is clearly exemplified in the work of the French philosopher and his-torian, Michel Foucault. Poststructuralists such as Foucault are concerned with *de*-constructing the concepts by which we have come to understand the human subject, including concepts such as 'the self', 'the social' and 'citizenship'.

Poststructuralists adopt a unique kind of deconstructive and analytic approach, with a specific purpose in mind. Because they seek to challenge the humanist notion of an unchanging human nature, they favour a historical method which sees different forms of consciousness and identities as historically produced. The method of genealogy, proposed by Foucault, has been the method adopted by poststructuralists for disrupting the certainties of the present and allowing new perspectives to emerge, including those of previously marginalised groups (see Chapter 2). Poststructuralists challenge the notion that there is an overall pattern in history and that the present state of affairs is inevitable and immutable. Given poststructuralists' scepticism about grand theory building and the claim of positivistic science to know all there is to know, it is not surprising that poststructural work has also tended to focus on the mundane, everyday practices which constitute our social realities. Their focus on 'subjugated' and 'disqualified' knowledges tends to place them in sharp opposition to the sociological tradition (from Marx, Durkheim and Weber to the present) that privilenges professional knowledge over the lay interpretation of reality (Best 1994: 44). This is not to say that they have abandoned analysis of broader social structures or of the broader sweeps of history, or eschew the use of systematic methods. However, the historical and social determinism of structuralist sociology is rejected in favour of an analysis of the interconnections between the macro-level and the micro-level workings of power, particularly as these are played out in specific domains, for example, in the workplace, in education and in the clinic, and how this affects our understandings of the human subject and people's awareness of themselves as subjects (i.e. their subject-ivities). Some of these features of poststructuralism are ones which are also often associated with postmodernism.

The term poststructuralism is sometimes used interchangeably with postmodernism, and this is also the source of some confusion. This is not to say that poststructuralism is unrelated to post-modernism. However, the exact nature of the relationship depends upon one's particular conception of postmodernism, that is, whether one is using this term to refer to a period in history, a cultural context or a theoretical approach. Poststructuralism has been variously described as a symptom of the postmodern culture which it seeks to describe, as a part of the maxtrix of postmodern theory, and as a discourse of and about modernism (see Dickens and Fontana 1994: 89–90; Best and Kellner 1991: 25; Huyssen 1984: 39, in Smart 1993). These definitions highlight the significance of the broader cultural and theoretical context within which post-structuralism emerges and with which poststructuralists engage. However, they also tend to convey the impression that there has been an abrupt and absolute shift in culture and theory which has not in fact occurred. The popularisation of the ideas of writers such as Baudrillard, who portrays the present age as one in which the distinction between reality and illusion has disappeared – where what is real is but a simulacrum and where 'the social' no longer exists – and Lyotard, whose highly influential book *The Postmodern Condition* (1984) provides a polemic attack against the discourses of modernity while offering new postmodern positions, has had the unfortunate effect of suggesting that there has been an abrupt break with the past. The very use of the prefix 'post' in poststructuralism and postmodernism indeed suggests a radical shift in perspective or milieu that has often been used by critics to dismiss the contributions of those scholars who draw on poststructural or postmodern ideas. Although poststructuralism has emerged in a context of significant change – one in which the very foundations of knowledge are being questioned – it is important to recognise continuities as well as ruptures in our ways of thinking about the social world. For instance, the particular concept of 'the social' that has underpinned thinking about social policy and social action for much of the last two hundred years continues to predominate, despite its erosion under neo-liberalism (see Chapter 4). Faith in rational science and in the ability to manage or ameliorate social problems rationally also endures in diverse areas of culture, including the policy arena, where professional, science-based knowledge and 'top-down' approaches to formulating policy continue to hold a privileged position *vis-à-vis* non-professional or lay knowledge and 'bottom-up' approaches. Thus, while contemporary societies are undergoing changes of a kind and order that call for novel approaches, we need to guard against setting up false dichotomies of 'old' and 'new' or 'past' and 'present' and hence overlooking the importance of continuities in our 'ways of seeing'.

One of our intentions has been to present our arguments in a way which allows conflicts in viewpoint and unresolved dilemmas of theory to emerge. Although we share certain concerns and can agree on the broad outlines of poststructuralism and how it might contribute to policy analysis, there are also many points on which we disagree and arguments which need further thought. We each make use of and engage with poststructural ideas in somewhat different ways. As you will note, each of the chapters is followed by short reflexive essays which constitute responses by each of us to queries raised by the others to our argument. This gives the book more of an interactive flavour than is found in most other texts. We hope that these essays serve as a pedagogic device, helping to convey to students, and to lecturers not familiar with poststructuralist thought, the challenges posed by poststructuralism to the idea of the authoritative voice. In organising the material in this way, we hope to stimulate further debate, rather than to foreclose discussion about the contributions of poststructural analysis to policy analysis.

The relationship between poststructuralism and the social policy literature

What is the relationship between poststructuralism and the social policy literature? In order to answer this question properly, we need first to clarify what we mean when we refer to the 'social policy tradition'. A useful way of doing this is by contrast: that is, by establishing which kinds of policy writing are *not* part of the social policy tradition as we understand it.

We start with those texts which aim to provide a set of strategic or analytical tools for the practitioner (thus, for example, Hogwood and Gunn's *Policy Analysis for the Real World* (1984)). Typically, such texts deal with the formulation, implementation and evaluation of policy. Their substantive concerns include the nature of decision making, the means of forecasting and diagnosing policy issues and the locus of policy making. Questions relating to the operation of power and the nature of the state are rarely raised. The social and political policy context is a *given*, something which the intelligent policy maker takes into account and deals with as he or she designs and implements chosen strategies.

In contrast, the social policy tradition (in both its more orthodox and critical forms) has such issues at the heart of its concerns. It sets out to describe the social, economic and political conditions in which policy arises. Social policy research aims to provide a critical understanding of how policy is made and what its effects are. Epsing-Anderson's *Welfare States in Transition* (1996) provides a recent example. Its writings are intended to inform the work of the practitioner but not to provide a set of instructions and are intended for academics as well as policy makers.

The social policy tradition also needs to be distinguished from *public policy* writing. This distinction operates at two levels: *area* and *perspective*. As far as area is concerned, public policy texts typically deal with a broad range of policies including macro and micro economic reform, industrial relations, transport, the environment, health, education and (less often) welfare. In contrast, social policy texts generally restrict themselves to areas more obviously linked to the welfare state: health, education, income security and employment are the prime examples. In relation to perspective, public policy writings focus on the institutional settings of political decision making, the actual operations of power and the influence of interest groups, while social policy writings centre on the normative bases and distributional consequences of particular policies.[1] (This difference is only an approximation, given the variety of writings in each school.)

Our book is primarily devoted to 'social' policy areas in that three chapters deal with the established trio: health, education and welfare. Its perspective, though, departs from both 'public' and 'social' policy orientations as described above. It is, we have claimed, 'poststructural'. How does this affect our approach to policy? In what ways are poststructural approaches different from what went before? And, in particular, given the focus of this book, how do 'poststructural' perspectives differ from 'social policy' perspectives?

Before attempting to answer these questions, a word of caution. In proposing an (approximate) distinction between 'poststructural' and 'social policy' perspectives, we do not claim to have entered a whole different genre of writing. Proponents of new schools tend to overemphasise the distinctiveness of their own approach and dwell at some length on the deficiencies of what went before. Poststructuralism has been no exception to this (cf. Garland 1997). In contrast, we suggest that it is important to emphasise continuities alongside differences, and to acknowledge sameness as well as contrast, and dialogue as well as opposition. In this context, we draw attention to three important characteristics shared by poststructural and established social policy perspectives.

First, both belong to a *critical* tradition in that they query/reformulate/disestablish current certainties and operations. Both perspectives know that apparently progressive measures may have divisive and oppressive effects. This, as Mann (1998) points out, is as true of Titmuss as of many of the newer poststructural or 'postmodern' approaches to policy. Second, both tend to share a *leftist* position in that they are concerned with the ways in which current patterns of power and knowledge operate to disenfranchise and silence certain groups of people and/or ways of thinking. The language may have changed but the direction of the critique is similar. Third, both share a *social* orientation, in that the terms and conditions under which the public domain is organised is a central problematic for both. Given these continuities, what are the main differences between 'poststructural' and 'social policy' perspectives?

One of the most frequently cited distinctions relates to the place which a normative position plays in the analysis. On this line of reasoning, a social policy perspective is more likely to have an up-front normative stance and be directed towards achieving a specific normative project, be that Marxist, feminist, Fabian, social democratic or anarchist. In contrast, poststructural approaches are said to be directed towards explicating the characteristics of current policies rather than voicing a particular normative position (cf. O'Malley *et al.* 1997). While we accept the general direction of this argument (and revoice it at various points in the book), we suggest that it cannot be taken too far. It both exaggerates the extent to which established social policy texts set out to promulgate a particular normative perspective[2] and masks the normativity invested in poststructuralist accounts. Explication and prescription are invariably interwoven.

There are other, perhaps more promising, ways of distinguishing between 'social policy' and 'poststructural' perspectives. These relate to the construction of the state, the status of general categories and the notion of 'truth' (cf. Hillyard and Watson 1996).

Social policy accounts generally treat the state as a unitary object which has its own rationale, motivations and interests. Such a notion is encapsulated in references to the 'capitalist', 'patriarchal' or 'democratic' state. In such accounts, the positioning of the state – whether it is partisan, a site of struggle or a court of appeal – varies, but the idea of it as some kind of 'thing' which thinks and responds persists. In contrast, poststructural narratives dismember the state, emphasising the various and inconsistent practices which shape its manifold components.

The position of the state as the main seat of power is correspondingly down-played in poststructuralist approaches. It emerges as one segment of a much broader play of power relations involving professionals, bureaucracies, schools, families, leisure organisations and so forth. In Foucault's terms, the various institutions and practices of the state operate as part of a 'capillary' of relations in which power continually circulates and recirculates. Accordingly, poststructural interest is as much directed to the local dole office as the central policy making bureau, and to the doctor's surgery or social worker's office as the Departments of Health and Welfare.

The general categories which characterise many social policy accounts are dislodged in poststructural analysis. Notions of 'class', 'gender' and 'race' are problematised in so far as they represent undifferentiated categories which explain the genesis of 'capitalist', 'patriarchal' or 'racist' policies. It is, though, important not to overemphasise the difference between social policy and poststructural accounts as far as this is concerned. Social policy texts, particularly feminist ones, have long acknowledged the need to dislodge global categories and explore the interconnections between gender, class, race, age, differential ability, etc. (for example, Williams 1985). And poststructural approaches, in their turn, deploy general categories in certain circumstances and for certain defined purposes.[3] What differentiates poststructural accounts from social policy approaches is that the notion of difference provides the *starting point* of analysis rather than something which is acknowledged to exist within a prior category.

Questions relating to the status of 'truth' and its displacement in postenlightenment thought have been extensively discussed elsewhere. They are the main concern of antifoundationalist writers such as Rorty (1989) and Bernstein (1991). We shall not attempt to canvass these debates but simply signal their implications for poststructural accounts of policy. We need to start with a disclaimer. Critical policy accounts have not, in fact, taken 'truth' as given. Quite the contrary: interrogations from Marx on have accepted the connection between ruling interests and ruling ideas. In this sense, Foucaultian ideas about the interconnection between knowledge and power are scarcely new. What *is* relatively new is Foucault's insistence on the *indivisibility* of knowledge and power: 'we are subjected to the production of truth through power, and we cannot exercise power except through the production of truth' (Foucault 1980: 93). This means that there is no free domain, no possibility of uttering truth outside an ambit of power relations.

This has significant implications for poststructural approaches to social policy. First, and least contentiously, it consistently directs our attention to the relationship between knowledge and power: in this instance, to the relationship between expert knowledges of the economy, health, families, education and so forth and the kinds of political and social programmes to which these knowledges give rise. This interest is exemplified throughout the chapters of this book.

Second, it means that universal symbols and promises – 'socialism', 'social justice', the 'collective good' – are ruled out of court. As well as being related to the relativisation of truth, the disappearance of these universals is directly connected to the post-structural emphasis on difference. To the extent that social life is characterised by multiple and incommensurable sites and subject positions, it becomes difficult to talk of collective goals, of the public good or of any universal notion of social justice. It is at this point that poststructural analysis runs into serious difficulty. In the eyes of some critics at least, poststructuralism not only fails to oppose the atomisations of neo-liberal policies but actually reproduces its individualistic assumptions (cf. Taylor-Gooby 1994). The charge merits further consideration.

Poststructural analysis, neo-liberalism and the fragmentation of the public domain

As already pointed out in this Introduction, neo-liberal policies have weakened and fractured the public domain through privatising, contracting out, downsizing, rationing and disestablishing a host of public services and utilities. The political rationality which accompanies and justifies these moves not only speaks of restraint but also of its mission to recognise and reward individual choice and personal decision making (Rose 1992, 1993, 1996).

Neo-liberal rationalities are popular political discourses and thus a quite different beast from academic poststructural analyses. They also form the *subject* of much poststructural analysis, particularly as far as the governmentality literature is concerned. And much poststructural analysis is devoted to dislodging the certainties of neo-liberal orthodoxies. Is it nevertheless true that poststructural analysis is debarred from assisting in the reconstruction of a public sphere precisely because of its own insistence on multiplicity and difference?

Any answer to this question must first clarify the way in which neo-liberal and poststructural discourses actually deploy the notion of 'difference'. Neo-liberal usages commonly refer to the separate interests of indivisible human actors: that is, to the rational calculations of the 'economic man' who stands at the centre of liberal thought. In contrast, poststructural accounts deploy 'difference' to refer to the multiplicity of subject positions produced through the operations of power/knowledge: positions which constantly shift, are differentially experienced by people, and cannot be traced back, or reduced, to any single actor.

Building on its notion of difference, and on its armoury of beliefs more generally, neo-liberalism perceives a 'truth' towards which its energies should be directed: the promotion of personal choice and individual enterprise. This leads to a clear if limited role for the state: it is to be devoted to the central administration of resources, the devolution of management, the maintenance of law and order and – usually but not invariably – the protection of moral standards. Poststructural accounts, with their interest in the circulation of power around and beyond the official institutions of the central state, are able to take a different view of the relationship between state and society. There is no necessary antagonism between 'state' and 'society' and, indeed, no necessary distinction in the first place. This provides the space for an attempt to articulate the political conditions which would variously assist citizens to be involved in their own governance at a local as well as a central level. In this way, poststructuralist accounts can, we suggest, assist in the reconstruction of the public domain, even if in an altered form. We refer briefly to two main types of theorising.[4]

First, there are a group of writers, influenced by poststructuralist thinking and loyal to older democratic concerns, who argue for a genuine devolution of decision making power combined with an adequate guaranteed minimum income (GMI) or citizens income (CI). The aim here is to disperse the locales of power and provide the conditions under which local networks of 'thick welfare, thin collectivism' may emerge. Paul Hirst's *Associative Democracy* (1994) provides the best-known example. Such an approach could provide a different relationship between civil society and the local state and undermine the dualisms on which that distinction has historically rested (Hoggett and Thompson 1998). It does, however, tend to operate at a level of abstraction which ignores the actual practicalities of policy making, particularly as far as distributional issues are concerned.

Second, there is a second group of theorists who, true to their poststructural affiliations, are reluctant to prescribe outcomes or political programmes in any detail. Instead of speaking of the public good or even the public domain, such writers consider the kind of democratic conditions which would acknowledge contestation and promote the expression of difference. The interlocking although differentiated nature of social and political life is recognised and a plea made for an environment which allows people to live together without claiming to 'know' or 'speak for' each other. Writers in this genre aim to promote mutuality rather than insist on solidarity. In this vein, Iris Young (1990, 1993) argues that the notion of community with its tendency to 'subsume and delimit difference' should be replaced by the ideal of 'the unoppressive city' as a space which allows for 'unassimilated otherness' (Hillyard and Watson 1996: 336). Citizenship, in short, is to be promoted as an expression of openness, tolerance, difference and mutuality rather than sameness. Such themes are developed by Fraser (1994, 1995), Frazer and Lacey (1993), Phillips (1993) and Yeatman (1994).

While we do not directly discuss these writings in this book, citizenship, and its relationship to neo-liberalism, is one of our key themes and so we should, therefore, at the outset clarify our assumptions about citizenship. First, however, we feel it is necessary to provide a brief review of the broader economic and political context giving rise to neo-liberal rationalities and policies.

The economic and political context

The period between 1945 and the early 1970s was a period of economic stability and prosperity for western nations. Often referred to as the Long Boom, this Keynesian/Fordist settlement between capital and labour, of mass production and mass consumption was reinforced and supported by welfare state provisions. The character of the welfare state varied according to the specifics of the national circumstances and traditions – thus the Beveridge model of the UK welfare state and the Australian 'workers' welfare state' (Castles 1988) each reflected the cultural and political assumptions of their particular societies. In each case, the objectives of public policy were broadly, to ensure 'the general maximization of welfare within a *national* society' (Cerny 1990: 205; emphasis added). However, over the decade or so between the early 1970s and the early 1980s, this Keynesian/Fordist compromise unravelled as a result of the collapse of the Bretton Woods international monetary system; the oil crisis of the Organization of Petroleum Exporting Countries (OPEC) and the subsequent oil price rises; the internationalisation of financial markets and the abolition of exchange rate controls; 'reindustrialisation'; the rise, particularly in Asia, of the newly industrialised countries (the NICs); pressures for free trade and market deregulation; and new post-Fordist models of flexible production (Hirst and Thompson 1996: 5). Together with the ensuing inflation and elevated levels of unemployment (particularly long-term unemployment) in the western industrialised countries, these resulted in new international economic and trading relations.

The late twentieth century has also been characterised by changing patterns of production. The nationally based mechanised assembly-line manufacture of Fordist mass production has been challenged by post-Fordist models of more flexible production, niche marketing and niche manufacturing. This is a model of 'tailoring' production more closely to the demands of international competition, and is based on developments in computer technologies, laser technologies, communications technologies and the like. Moreover, production is increasingly global: components are manufactured and/or assembled in factories and plants located in different world locations.

This new economy is claimed to be dominated by multinational companies (MNCs) and transnational companies (TNCs) whose investment decisions are influenced by principles of efficiency and productivity, rather than by national loyalties. This is the context of globalisation consisting of 'a *global auction* for investment, technology and jobs' where 'the prosperity of workers will depend on an ability to trade their skills, knowledge and entrepreneurial acumen in an unfettered global market place' (Brown and Lauder 1996: 2–3).

Globalisation is a narrative of incorporation into a world system. The central premise of this narrative is the new world order of a truly global economy. The new global order is argued to be the culmination of a number of interdependent developments which include:

- the aspirations of virtually all societies throughout the world towards western materialist/consumer-based lifestyles;
- the penetration and near hegemony throughout the world of western popular culture, and particularly American expressions of this mass culture;
- the increasing dominance of western, and particularly US sourced models of production and consumption;
- the increasing integration of world economies into a single global international market;
- free trade and the new international division of labour.

Late twentieth-century communications technologies, together with the post Cold War peace – what Fukuyama (1993) has called 'the end of history' – both facilitate and provide a context for processes of globalisation. Whilst globalisation ostensibly has cultural, political and economic dimensions, all of the above developments are structured by a rationality which is principally western and principally economic. Although the global culture which our increasing communications capacities is shaping appears to be principally social, it is a culture of mass consumption. It is hence ineluctably articulated into western capitalism and global markets.

The claim of globalisation is that national economies are being increasingly subsumed into a global economy, so that the discipline of international markets and money markets should determine public policy rather than national, social and/or political priorities. These policies, almost without exception, require states to reduce public spending, deregulate capital and labour markets, minimise welfare provision and either eliminate or privatise as much as possible of the welfare state.

Brown and Lauder (1996) posit two 'ideal type' economic responses to the new conditions of economic globalisation: neo-Fordism (or the New Right) and post-Fordism (which Brown and Lauder term 'Left Moderniser'). These loosely correspond to demand-side and supply-side approaches respectively. Neo-Fordism is characterised by emphases on markets, labour market 'flexibility' (through lower labour costs), efficiency (enhancing productivity through minimising production costs), deregulation, privatisation and managerialism; whereas post-Fordism is a 'high skill/high wage' route to national prosperity and is characterised by high skill, high value added innovative production and market flexibility through multiskilling.

In response to the changing economic circumstances of globalisation, the state may be actively interventionist – a strategic player attempting, through labour market policies and education and training, to facilitate the development of a high-wage, high-skill post-Fordist economy. Alternatively, the state can adopt the *laissez-faire*, minimalist neo-Fordist strategy of leaving economic restructuring to market forces. Whatever the strategy/approach, the objective remains international competitiveness in global capitalist markets. From the late 1980s, Australian Labor governments adopted the active strategic route to economic prosperity, attempting to stimulate the development of a high-skill, high-wage economy of the kind envisaged by Robert Reich in his influential book *The Work of Nations*. Since the election of the conservative Liberal–National Party Coalition government in 1996, Australian public policy, particularly labour market policies, have been dominated and structured according to neo-Fordist principles and assumptions. In contrast, UK public policy has moved from the neo-Fordism characteristic of the Thatcher years to the post-Fordism – or 'Left Moderniser' strategies – of New Labour.

The mixed economy and welfare states of the post Second World War period have been replaced by what Cerny (1990: 204–32) calls 'the competition state'. In the competition state, society and the economy are conflated, and an economic rationality is the discursive foundation organising social relations. Cerny (ibid.: 205) describes the transition from the welfare state to the competition state as follows:

> a shift in the focus of [state] intervention from the development of a range of 'strategic' or 'basic' industries . . . to one of flexible response to competitive market conditions in a range of diversified and rapidly evolving international marketplaces . . . [and] a shift in the focal point of party and governmental politics from the general maximization of welfare within a national society (full employment, redistributive transfers and social service provision) to the promotion of enterprise, innovation and profitability in both private and public sectors.

Under welfare state conditions the state's role was 'to *take certain activities out of the market place* . . . and to "socialize" them'. Whereas the welfare state was a '*decommodifying* agent', the competition state is a '*commodifying* agent' (ibid.: 230).

The economic priorities of the competition state apply not only to the objective of competitiveness in the increasingly open and integrated environment of international capitalism, but operate also to reconfigure relations within the state. Competition is thus a national imperative 'requiring' efficiency, privatisation and corporatisation in the public sector – for example Australia's National Competition Policy (which resulted from the Hilmer Report of 1993) requires that governments must ensure 'competitive neutrality' with private sector providers of services or divest themselves of activities 'more appropriately' serviced by private industry. In addition, the competitive individualism of neo-liberal thought and market relations becomes the normative paradigm for social relations – the freedom of individuals is the freedom to engage via contractual relations. It is in this context that the notion of citizenship has increasingly been contested.

The concept of citizenship

As mentioned, 'citizenship' is a major recurring theme in our book. Over the past decade in Australia, as elsewhere, there has been a resurgence of interest in the idea of citizenship both in academia and in public life more generally. The notion of citizenship has been taken up by public intellectuals, think tanks, research centres, academic journals, educational reformers, as well as by politicians and government agencies. In 1994, in Australia, the then Keating Labor Government commissioned a 'civics expert group' to come up with recommendations about the best ways to promote a greater awareness of civic life (Civic Experts Group 1994). The Howard Coalition Government has also deployed the rhetoric of active citizenship, particularly in relation to deflecting opposition to its reduced support for health, education and welfare services and the redirection of education towards more explicitly economic goals (Kemp 1997).

The immediate catalyst for the resurgence of interest in citizenship has of course been the ascendancy of neo-liberalism, or economic rationalism as it is known in Australia (Mouffe 1988; Meredyth 1997). The rise of the New Right has meant the progressive dismantling of the taken-for-granted postwar social democratic/welfare state policy framework (though not by any means a withdrawal of strategic control of social life). The changing economic and political circumstances associated with the end of Fordism and the increasing globalisation of economic life has made it extremely difficult to rebuild effective political support for the old social democratic framework. Instead, socialists, social democrats, feminists, radical environmentalists and social liberals have drawn on the language of citizenship, civic life and civil society as a way of resisting the economistic assault on social life and public institutions (Cox 1995; Marsh 1995; Pixley 1993). In the context of the reduction of public services, the privatisation of public life and the foregrounding of public choice theories of public policy, all in the name of the imperative of increasing global competitiveness, the idea of citizenship offers a new/old language to defend the distinctive and irreducibly political nature of civic life.

An important aspect of this revival of civic discourse has been a renewed interest in T.H. Marshall's account of the historical expansion of the legal, political and social rights (Bulmer and Rees 1996; King and Waldron 1988). However, just as significant has been the recovery of an older civic republican (and, for some, communitarian) tradition of citizenship (Barber 1984; Beiner 1995; Mouffe 1988, 1992; Oldfield 1990; Turner 1990), a tradition which differs in a number of important ways from liberal conceptions of citizenship. According to the new civic republicans, citizenship should be understood as not just a legal status or a set of rights associated with (passive) membership of a nation-state but a responsibility for active civic involvement in community affairs and public life. It should also entail notions of political learning and the development of shared conceptions of the common good, rather than merely the pursuit of preformed interests or the defence of individual rights. It should express a rather different conception of the relationship between public and private spheres. Furthermore, in the view of people such as Bellah, Boyte, Gamson and Putnam, the rich civic life of an associational civil society is the necessary precondition for both good government and a prosperous economy.

Although for some on the left, civic republican ideas of civil society and citizenship provide the best prospect for the defence of the social against neo-liberal 'reform', others are not so sure (Mouffe 1988; Young 1989). Social democrats and feminists worry about what the implications might be of civic republicanism, particularly its notion of the common good and the expectation of active participation, for the achievements of modernity: personal freedoms, individual rights, social diversity and confessional pluralism. A lively debate continues, particularly in North America, over the relevance and desirability of a civic republican ideal of citizenship.

Meanwhile, at a more pragmatic level, another problematic aspect of the notion of active citizenship is its effective cooption by neo-liberal regimes. By urging citizens to take a more active responsibility for matters of distributive justice, environmental care and so on, governments seek to reduce public expectations with respect to state provision for health, education and welfare provision. In this perspective, the notion of active citizenship becomes much more politically ambiguous, able to express either a communitarian ideal of social solidarity and community or a neo-liberal vision of a minimalist state and a renewed ethos of voluntary self-help.

However, from a poststructuralist perspective, such debates are, first, much too abstract and removed from the detailed circumstances of people's everyday lives, and, second, fail to recognise the ways in which the notions of citizenship are deployed within those political rationalities through which populations are governed and self-governed. Burchell (1995) argues that both sides of the current debates about citizenship reflect the continuing influence of a post-Rousseauian political philosophy, and both assume one or other sort of a transcendental moral subject. Burchell (ibid.: 549) comments:

> What is altogether missing from this kind of controversy is a sense of the citizen as a social creation, as a historical *persona*, whose characteristics have been developed in particular times and places through the activities of social discipline, both externally on the part of governments and 'internally' by techniques of self-discipline and self-formation.

One of the tasks of the chapters in this book is to explore the ways in which the language of citizenship is being deployed within the discourses of neo-liberal governance in the context of specific social sites, and the ways in which these discourses are involved in the formation of particular subjectivities and political identities. The primary aim is to render visible the rationalities of governance which remain largely unrecognised in current debates about citizenship and to notice more restrictive meanings of citizenship that are produced. As Patricia Harris comments, in so doing, a poststructuralist analysis makes it possible to open up the points of tension and conflict, or the 'lines of fault' within the governing neo-liberal rationality.

The chapters in this book explore the language of citizenship within a governing neo-liberal discourse in the context of four crucial social sites: the provision of social welfare; the application of new forms of genetic diagnosis; the reform of higher education in Britain and Australia; and the more general diffusion of technological innovation in everyday life. Whilst the focus of these discussions is primarily diagnostic rather than condemnatory (O'Malley *et al.* 1997: 260), they do make visible the essentially contested nature of the idea of citizenship. By bringing into focus the ways in which neo-liberal governance gives rise to specific practices and subjectivities, these chapters also illuminate the interplay between subjects and the larger rationalities in which they are located (van Krieken 1996).

Outline of the chapters

In Chapter 2, Patricia Harris examines the ways in which the changing rationalities of liberal governance have constructed the subject within the specific contexts of public welfare provision. She locates the current regime of advanced liberal governance in the context of earlier regimes of classical and expansive liberal governance. In her account advanced liberalism has had a threefold effect on a sense of social order: in terms of a new contractualism, the fragmentation of the social, and the 'degovernmentalisation of the state itself'. Despite this, advanced liberalism is not so much a radical departure from the tradition as the refurbishment of older forms of governance which located subjects in a state of welfare dependency.

In her view, it is unlikely that the diffusion of the governing rationality of advanced liberalism can be sustained without generating opposition and increasing social resistance. In her chapter, she discusses the possible alternative rationalities which might enable the recovery of the social. On the one hand, she does not want to abandon the more inclusive, universalising ideas of justice within the socialist tradition but, on the other, she insists on the need to recognise the 'multiplicity of justice claims'.

In Chapter 3, Janice Dudley explores the concept of active citizenship in the context of the reform of higher education policy in Australia and the UK. Through an analysis of the West and Dearing reports, which have framed higher education policy debates in the two countries, she shows how the language of citizenship, participation and responsibility, as well as the key metaphor, 'learning for life', articulates the rationality of rule of advanced liberalism or neo-liberalism. She suggests that the ambiguities in the meanings of citizenship in this neo-liberal discourse also creates possibilities for resistance: that the ideas of empowerment, although part of the lexicon of neo-liberal regulation, might none the less generate subversive alternatives.

In Chapter 4, Alan Petersen develops a similar exploration of the ways in which the idea of the responsible subject is articulated within the emerging practices of genetic-based public health. Here the development of new techniques for the diagnosis of genetic diseases generates new kinds of risk and new responsibilities for 'governing one's own genetic fate'. Alan argues that by recognising the tensions between lay 'rationalities' and expert rationalities, the new genetics has the potential to become an important site for contesting citizenship.

In Chapter 5, Ian Barns explores the connections between citizenship and the diffusion of new technologies. He notes that one of the curious features of the debate over citizenship has been the relative lack of attention to the discursive significance of technologies. Drawing on constructivist and cultural-hermeneutical approaches to technology, he argues that, whilst at the level of everyday practice technologies make possible a range of possible interpretations, at the level of techno-economic systems and a broader epistemological or discursive framework, the broader trajectory of technological innovation is towards an increasing commodification and disenchantment of experience. Finally, he briefly explores the moral/spiritual possibilities of a more reflexive subjectivity within a technological environment.

Finally, in Chapter 6, we draw together the main themes of the book and raise the question of how the more critical understanding of citizenship afforded by poststructuralism might be useful to people involved in the policy process as policy makers, as policy activists or as citizens. The chapter is based on an edited transcript of an audio-taped discussion among Alan, Ian, Janice and Patricia exploring the ways in which the language of 'citizenship' can be developed as a language of resistance and/or of governance in each of the four major areas of policy covered in the chapters.

Notes

1   This division of labour both disguises the 'social' aspects of economic and industrial domains and fails to give sufficient attention to the political processes through which various 'social' agendas are hammered out. In this context, a more helpful approach is provided by Bell and Head (1994) in their *State, Economy and Public Policy in Australia*.

2   While some writers in the social policy tradition have been concerned to promote a particular position (thus, for example, Galper 1980 and Gough 1979), others have concentrated on revealing patterns of inequality and oppression without necessarily promulgating a specific political allegiance (e.g. Williams 1985).

3   This point is argued by Patricia Harris (this volume) in response to a question posed by Alan Petersen.

4   We do not include the kind of solution offered by Anthony Giddens (1994) here. Giddens calls for a 'positive' form of welfare which emphasises the quality of life, social groupings, local ties and self-identity, and downplays class, production, redistribution and material possession. We exclude Giddens because his analysis is not 'poststructural' even though it does deal with certain 'postmodern' concerns.

References

Barber, B. (1984) *Strong Democracy: Participatory Politics for a New Age*, Berkeley, CA: University of California Press.

Beiner, R. (ed.) (1995) *Theorizing Citizenship*, New York: SUNY.

Bell, S. and Head, B. (1994) *State, Economy and Public Policy in Australia*, Oxford: Oxford University Press.

Bernstein, R. (1991) *The New Constellation: The Ethical-Political Horizons of Modernity/Postmodernity*, Cambridge: Polity Press.

Best, S. (1994) 'Foucault, postmodernism, and social theory', in D.R. Dickens and A. Fontana (eds), *Postmodernism and Social Inquiry*, London: UCL Press.

Best, S. and Kellner, D. (1991) *Postmodern Theory: Critical Interrogations*, New York: Guilford Press.

Boyte, H. and Kari, N. (1996) *Building America: The Democratic Promise of Public Work*, Philadelphia: Temple University Press.

Brown, P. and Lauder, H. (1996) 'Education, globalization and economic development', *Journal of Education Policy*, 11, 1: 1–26.

Bulmer, M. and Rees, A.M. (eds) (1996) *Citizenship Today: The Contemporary Relevance of T.H. Marshall*, Bristol, PA: UCL Press.

Burchell, D. (1995) 'The attributes of citizens: virtue, manners and the activity of citizenship', *Economy and Society*, 24, 4: 540–8.

Castles, F. (1988) *Australian Public Policy and Economic Vulnerability*, St Leonards, Sussex: Allen and Unwin.

Cerny, P.G. (1990) *The Changing Architecture of Politics: Structure, Agency, and the Future of the State*, London: Sage.

Civic Experts Group (1994) *Whereas the People . . . Civic and Citizenship Education: Report of Civic Experts Group*, Canberra: Australian Government Publishing Service.

Cox, E. (1995) *A Truly Civil Society*, the 1995 Boyer Lectures, Sydney: ABC Books.

Dickens, D.R. and Fontana, A. (eds) (1994) *Postmodernism and Social Inquiry*, London: UCL Press.

Epsing-Anderson, G. (1996) *Welfare States in Transition*, London: Sage.

Foucault, M. (1980) 'Two lectures', in C. Gordon (ed.) *Power/Knowledge: Selected Interviews and Other Writings*, New York: Pantheon Books.

Fraser, N. (1994) 'Re-thinking the public sphere: a contribution to the critique of actually existing democracy', in H.A. Giroux and P.L. Mclaren (eds), *Between Borders: Pedagogy and the Politics of Cultural Studies*, London: Routledge.

Fraser, N. (1995) 'Politics, culture and the public sphere: toward a postmodern conception', in L. Nicholson and S. Seidman (eds), *Social Postmodernism: Beyond Identity Politics,* Cambridge: Cambridge University Press.

Frazer, E. and Lacey, N. (1993) *The Politics of Community: A Feminist Critique of the Liberal-Communitarian Debate,* Hemel Hempstead, Herts: Harvester.

Fukuyama, F. (1993) *The End of History and the Last Man,* New York: Avon Books.

Galper, J. (1980) *Social Work Practice: A Radical Perspective,* Englewood Cliffs, NJ: Prentice-Hall.

Garland, D. (1997) '"Governmentality" and the problem of crime', *Theoretical Criminology,* 1, 2: 173–214.

Giddens, A. (1994) *Beyond Left and Right,* Cambridge: Polity Press.

Gough, I. (1979) *The Political Economy of the Welfare State,* London: Macmillan.

Hillyard, P. and Watson, S. (1996). 'Postmodern social policy: a contradiction in terms?', *Journal of Social Policy,* 25, 3: 321–46.

Hilmer, F. (1993) *National Competition Policy,* Report of the Independent Committee of Inquiry into Competition Policy in Australia (the Hilmer Report), Canberra: Australian Government Publishing Service.

Hirst, P. (1994) *Associative Democracy: New Forms of Economic and Social Governance,* Cambridge: Polity Press.

Hirst, P. and Thompson, G. (1996) *Globalization in Question,* Cambridge: Polity Press.

Hoggett, P. and Thompson, S. (1998) 'The delivery of welfare: the associationist vision', in J. Carter (ed.), *Postmodernity and the Fragmentation of Welfare,* London and New York: Routledge.

Hogwood, B.W. and Gunn, L.A. (1984) *Policy Analysis for the Real World,* Oxford: Oxford University Press.

Huyssen, A. (1984) 'Mapping the postmodern', *New German Critique,* 33, Fall: 5–52.

Kemp, D. (1997) *Discovering Democracy: Civics and Citizenship Education. A Ministerial Statement by the Hon. Dr David Kemp,* Canberra: Department of Employment, Education, Training and Youth Affairs.

Kennedy, K. (ed.) (1996) *New Challenges for Civics and Citizenship Education,* Belconnen, A.C.T.: Australian Curriculum Studies Association.

King, D. and Waldron, J. (1988) 'Citizenship, social citizenship and the defence of welfare provision', *British Journal of Political Science,* 18: 415–43.

Kymlicka, W. and Norman, W. (1994) 'Return of the citizen: a survey of recent works on citizenship theory', *Ethics,* 104 (January): 352–81.

Lyotard, J.F. (1984) *The Postmodern Condition: A Report on Knowledge,* Minneapolis: Minnesota Press.

Mann, K. (1998) '"One step beyond": critical social policy in a "postmodern" Britain', in J. Carter (ed.), *Postmodernity and the Fragmentation of Welfare,* London and New York: Routledge.

Marquand, D. (1997) *The New Reckoning: Capitalism, States and Citizens*, Cambridge: Polity Press.

Marsh, I. (1995) *Beyond the Two Party System: Political Representation, Economic Competitiveness and Australian Politics*, Cambridge: Cambridge University Press.

Meredyth, D. (1997) 'Invoking citizenship: education, competence and social rights', *Economy and Society*, 26, 2: 273–95.

Mouffe, C. (1988) 'The civics lesson', *New Statesman and Society*, 1, 18: 28–30.

Mouffe, C. (ed.) (1992) *Dimensions of Radical Democracy: Pluralism, Citizenship, Community*, London: Verso.

Oldfield, A. (1990) *Citizenship and Community: Civic Republicanism and the Modern World*, London: Routledge.

O'Malley, P., Weir, R. and Shearing, C. (1997) 'Governmentality, criticism and politics', *Economy and Society*, 26, 4: 501–17.

Phillips, A. (1993) *Democracy and Difference*, Cambridge: Polity Press.

Pixley, J. (1993) *Citizenship and Employment: Investigating Post-industrial Options*, Melbourne: Cambridge University Press.

Reich, R.B. (1991) *The Work of Nations: Preparing Ourselves for Twenty-first Century Capitalism*, New York: Alfred A. Knopf.

Rorty, R. (1989) *Contingency, Irony and Solidarity*, Cambridge: Cambridge University Press.

Rose, N. (1992) 'Governing the enterprising self', in P. Heelas and M. Morris (eds), *The Values of the Enterprise Culture: The Moral Debate*, London: Unwin Hyman.

Rose, N. (1993) 'Government, authority and expertise in advanced liberalism', *Economy and Society*, 22, 3: 283–327.

Rose, N. (1996) 'The death of the social', *Economy and Society*, 25, 3: 327–56.

Sarup, M. (1993) *An Introductory Guide to Poststructuralism and Postmodernism*, 2nd edn, Hemel Hempstead, Herts: Harvester Wheatsheaf.

Seidman, S. (ed.) (1996) *Queer Theory/Sociology*, Cambridge, MA: Blackwell.

Senate Standing Committee on Employment, Education and Training (1991) *Active Citizenship Revisited: A Report*, Canberra: Australian Government Publishing Service.

Smart, B. (1993) *Postmodernity*, London: Routledge.

Taylor-Gooby, P. (1994) 'Postmodernism and social policy: a great leap backwards?', *Journal of Social Policy*, 23, 3: 387–403.

Turner, B. (1990) 'Outline of a theory of citizenship', *Sociology*, 24, 2: 189–217.

van Krieken, R. (1996) 'Proto-governmentalization and the historical formation of organizational subjectivity', *Economy and Society*, 25, 2: 195–221.

Weedon, C. (1987) *Feminist Practice and Poststructuralist Theory*, Oxford: Blackwell.

Williams, F. (1985) *Social Policy: A Critical Introduction,* Cambridge: Polity Press.

Yeatman, A. (1994) *Postmodern Revisionings of the Political,* London: Routledge.

Young, I.M. (1989) 'Polity and group difference: a critique of the ideal of universal citizenship', *Ethics*, 99: 250–74.

Young, I.M. (1990) *Justice and the Politics of Difference,* Princeton, NJ: Princeton University Press.

Young, I.M. (1993) 'Together in difference: transforming the logic of group conflict', in J. Squires (ed.), *Principled Positions*, London: Harvester.

Chapter 2

Public welfare and liberal governance

Patricia Harris

Introduction

This chapter traces the ways in which western governments have responded to the historic fact that a significant proportion of their populations are prevented from earning income ('earning life') through the operations of the market. It discusses the terms and conditions on which economic support for low-income households has been provided over time and the political rationalities which have guided such provision. It draws on the arguments of certain Foucaultian theorists to suggest that governments' responses to their economically subject populations increasingly deploy a calculative type of welfare which divides citizens one from another. The notion of 'liberal governance' and the perceived relationship between 'dependent' and 'independent' populations are central to the analysis.

The theoretical literature associated with this kind of discussion draws from Foucault's work on governmentality, the focus of his interest in the late 1970s. Foucault's writings and lectures on governance represent a specific development of his earlier and more general ideas about power; they are complementary to, but not commensurate with, this interest. His insights into governmentality have been elaborated and extended by academics in Britain, Australia and, to a lesser extent, the United States. The writings of these theorists are extensively used in this chapter, which should be read as a synthesis or review rather than an original contribution to the literature.

Writings on governmentality seek to describe, explicate and understand the rationalities of governance rather than either to explain or to judge them. In the words of Barry *et al.* (1993: 260) they are 'concerned to diagnose the various forms of rationality that

govern our present rather than simply denounce or condemn them'.
In this respect, the governmentality literature follows the more
general Foucaultian reluctance to 'speak truth' or voice a totalising
explanation. The origins of this reluctance can be traced back to
certain aspects of French intellectual life in the 1960s. When scientific Marxism dismissed the student uprising of 1968 and the
widespread protests which followed as bourgeois revisionism,
Foucault questioned reductionist assumptions and called instead for
a form of inquiry which explored the micrological and manifold
channels through which power operates (Best and Kellner 1991:
23). With this, he rejected both the attempt to create a scientific
base for the study of social relations and any supposition that sociological thought could be guided by goals such as certainty, truth,
objectivity or liberation. In their place, he and others argued that
attention should be given to the specific relations between knowledge and power, the ways in which subjects are produced through
various forms of governance, and the 'conditions of possibility'
which underlie particular political rationalities. In the context of
this chapter, this means that we should be cautious of assuming
that public welfare has been designed to pacify the working class
or even that it is a product of class struggle – as variously argued
by, for example, Corrigan and Leonard (1978), Galper (1980),
Gough (1979) and Jones (1983). Instead, we need to explore the
various regimes of truth which lie behind the administration of
welfare programmes together with the social, political and economic
conditions which have made these programmes possible.

In Foucaultian terms this means that we adopt a 'genealogical'
type of inquiry. Genealogy explores the 'conditions and effects of
truth' (Dean 1992: 216). It involves a 'methodical problematisation
of the given' which is effected through:

> constituting lineages of those 'assemblages' – madness, crim-
> inality, sexuality, poverty, the economic, the social etc. – of
> which we are all too familiar, and which define the lineament
> of our present. Such assemblages are comprised of diverse and
> heterogeneous elements . . . [they] neither form an ideal unity,
> follow a smooth trajectory nor answer a determinative logic . . .
> genealogy emplaces the [findings of archaeology] as com-
> ponents in continuities without definite origin or end, and punc-
> tuated by events and ruptures.
>
> (Dean 1992: 216–17)

The refusal to evaluate and prescribe has led a number of critics to argue that the governmentality approach is inherently conservative. Under this view, the failure to take an explicitly normative position is tantamount to condoning the manifold injustices which characterise policy making and outcomes. Against this, it can be argued that the governmentality literature has the potential to destabilise existing orthodoxies, promote new ways of thinking about distribution and contestation, and generate a 'postsocialist' politics. Genealogical inquiry is important because it seeks to dislodge the certainties of the present. It allows us to question, for example, the notion that budgets are determined by 'economic necessity', that people should 'earn their living', and that productivity is to be demonstrated through paid work.

The extent to which this critical potential has been realised is, though, certainly arguable. Even proponents of governmentality acknowledge that the current literature falls significantly short of the critical ideals which informed Foucault's work (O'Malley *et al.* 1997). As Fraser (1981) suggested some time ago, Foucaultian theorists in general could be more prepared to acknowledge the normative premises which inform their work. If it is to be argued that genealogy has the power to dislodge existing certainties, then we should know what it is about those existing certainties that needs to be disrupted. Further, there is plenty of room to acknowledge the value of existing lines of critical inquiry. Contrary to what some of its advocates seem to imply, the governmentality approach should not be seen as a somehow 'better' form of inquiry from what went before. In particular, documenting welfare's unequal impact on people in relation to their class, gender, race or age (thus, for example, Bryson 1992; Wearing and Berreen 1994) remains, in my view, a central plank of any critical reform agenda. The governmentality approach is a complementary and not an alternative form of investigation to such accounts. Arguably, then, there is a need to make critique more explicit, more up-front.

The relationship between critique and explication is, however, complex. The earlier point, that we should be concerned to 'diagnose the various forms of rationality that govern our present rather than simply denounce or condemn them' (O'Malley *et al.* 1997: 260), still stands. Perhaps the best we can do to resolve the critique/ explication relationship at this stage is to voice two propositions simultaneously. First, we can suggest that our value position should not *determine* how we read and explain various political rationalities. Second, we can also acknowledge that critique is never-theless always/already *embedded in* explication: it resides, for example, in the very belief that genealogical inquiry aims to dislodge current certainties. Working with these two propositions simultaneously provides one with an *interactive* relationship between explication and critique in which each influences the other.

To some extent, the arrangement of material in this chapter reflects these suggestions. My reliance on the work of governmen-tality theorists ensures that the bulk of my discussion attempts to explicate rather than prescribe or judge. At the same time, I do provide an overt critique of current policies at the end of the chapter and periodic references to distributional issues throughout. Further, a more sustained critique informs the entire discussion. This is repre-sented in a consistent attempt to relativise – to 'render strange' – new and older truths about the market, welfare and independence. The normative position from which this chapter is written could best be described as broadly social democratic, underpinned by socialist and feminist concerns.

Before entering the substantive part of this discussion, some brief comments on the context of public welfare as a field of policy are in order.

The policy context of public welfare

Public welfare belongs to a broader range of income security policies, as Richard Titmuss (1963) makes clear. Titmuss argues that current welfare systems incorporate a range of programmes designed to safeguard people's financial situations and offset some of the unpredictabilities of the market. He designates three main categories of income support: 'fiscal welfare' (the provision of rebates and allowances through the taxation system); 'occupational welfare' (the provision of a range of benefits and allowances, including superannuation, through labour force participation); and 'public welfare' (the provision of income-tested pensions and bene-fits through the social security system). Titmuss goes on to say that the welfare system's capacity to protect the interests of higher-income earners is only revealed when all three components are taken into consideration.

His arguments reveal that assistance for low-income households is embedded in a matrix of programmes designed to protect the interests of the rich as well as provide some degree of security for the poor. Public welfare is part of the means whereby governments define and regulate the meaning and conditions of dependence and independence across multiple social and economic domains. Gender is deeply embedded in these strategic understandings, with women traditionally positioned as dependent on male breadwinners (Bryson 1992; Cass 1985; Wilson 1997). Because the economic subject is a male construct, the discourses surrounding public welfare have persistently assumed a set of labour force opportunities which characteristically accrue to men more than women. (This despite the fact that the number of women dependent on public welfare has historically been greater than the number of men.) The gendered nature of the rationalities which surround the governance of public welfare becomes evident later in this chapter. Official constructions of what counts as 'work' and the constitution of particular forms of 'independence' and 'enterprise' are particularly important in this context.

Public welfare, because it concerns support for populations defined as dependent, is problematic for liberal governance in a way in which fiscal and occupational welfare are not. From Poor Law on, assistance for dependent populations has simultaneously involved questions of autonomy/self-governance *and* dependence/ governmental intervention. In this respect, public welfare places liberal governance on the horns of a dilemma. On the one hand, the provision of economic support is necessary for the security and well-being of those unable to 'earn life' in the market. On the other hand, undue assistance, or assistance of the 'wrong' kind, may run counter to market processes and undermine the processes of 'natural self-regulation'. Similarly, the official desire to minimise abuse leads to various measures (restriction of movement, identity checks, behavioural scrutiny and so forth), and these measures may run counter to the more general principles of democracy and liberty. The ways in which these conflicting considerations have been juggled has undergone several changes over the last two centuries. Such changes reveal underlying shifts in the ways in which dependence and independence are constructed and managed under liberal governance.

It is the problematic nature of public welfare and the way it is managed which lie at the heart of this chapter. The rest of the discussion is organised in three parts. The first provides a review of some key terms used in the governmentality literature and sets out the framework for analysis in this chapter. It is designed for those who are not familiar with this work and can be skipped by those who are. The second section describes the ways in which western societies have managed the relations between dependent and independent populations over the past two centuries. The final part deals with the contemporary relationship between citizenship and public welfare and provides a critique of current arrangements.

Liberal governance: defining the field

Governing in a liberal way

In the Foucaultian literature the notion of 'government' is interpreted widely:

> Government must be allowed the very broad meaning which it had in the sixteenth century. 'Government' did not refer only to political structures or the management of states; rather it designated the way in which the conduct of individuals or states might be directed: the government of children, of souls, of communities, of families, of the sick. It did not cover only the legitimately constituted forms of political or economic subjection, but also modes of action, more or less considered and calculated, which were designed to act upon the possibilities of action of other people. To govern, in this sense, is to structure the possible field of action of others.
>
> (Foucault 1982: 221)

Under this definition, government is a set of on-going, more or less purposeful activities designed to direct behaviours and shape people's fortunes. These activities are by no means restricted to political governments or even the wider arena of the 'state'. They also incorporate statistical, professional, academic and commercial activities. As Dean (1992: 218) puts it, 'governance is a much broader term than the state, and in principle includes any relatively calculated practice of the direction of conduct, encompassing but not reducible to political government, to *the* government' (emphasis in the original).

Nevertheless, a special relationship exists between the practices of government and liberal-constitutional states. This is for two reasons. First, it appears that for the greater part of the nineteenth and twentieth centuries, governing practices have in fact come 'more and more under state control and influence' (Smart 1986: 162). Second, the activities of the state have themselves become increasingly involved with various calculations relating to the security of populations. It is in this vein that Smart (ibid.) speaks of a 'progressive governmentalisation of power relations' while Foucault suggests that 'what is really important for our modern times ... is not so much the state-domination of society, but the governmentalisation of the state' (Foucault 1991: 103). The reversal, or partial reversal, of these trends is discussed towards the end of this chapter.

The historical relationship between 'government' and the official practices of the state is sketched by Foucault (1991) in his brief discussion of the changing shape of ruling practices. Here he speaks about a certain 'mentality of government' ('governmentality') which has come to characterise western forms of governance from around the mid-eighteenth century on. Governmentality constitutes a 'very specific albeit complex form of power, which has as its target population, as its principal form of knowledge political economy, and as its technical means, apparatuses of security' (ibid.: 102). Its main purpose is not 'the act of government itself, but the welfare of the population, the improvement of its condition, the increase of its wealth, longevity, health etc.' (ibid.: 100).

This description of governmentality relies on a contrast with what went before: 'sovereignty' and 'discipline'. Foucault uses the term 'sovereignty' to refer to power designed to augment the status and possessions of the Prince. It was exemplified by the sixteenth and seventeenth-century administrative states and by a reliance on 'law' as an interdictory form of regulation (juridical monarchy). He talks of 'discipline' to mean power exercised directly over individuals in institutions such as prisons, schools and factories. It was designed to normalise, control and bring about conformity. Governmentality, with its focus on populations and their security, did not entirely supersede these two earlier forms of regulation. In Foucault's words:

> We need to see things not in terms of the replacement of a society of sovereignty by a disciplinary society and the subsequent replacement of a disciplinary society by a society of government; in reality one has a triangle, sovereign–discipline–government; which has as its primary target the population and as its essential mechanism the apparatuses of security.
>
> (Ibid.: 101)

This co-existence of governance, sovereignty and discipline is evident in the domain of public welfare where the governmental attempt to secure the fortunes of the population through the 'apparatuses of security' coincide both with the desire to protect the public purse and prevent abuse (sovereignty) and with direct measures to inspect and control recipients (discipline). This mixture of regulatory regimes, and the various political rationalities and technologies associated with them, repeatedly surfaces in this chapter.

Foucaultian writings on governance are writings about *western* governance. Notions of 'liberalism' play an important part in these discussions, with 'liberal' understood not as political philosophy but as a way of practising and thinking about government. Following Gordon (1991) and Rose (1996a), three key features of liberalism can be identified. First, liberal governance operates at arm's length from its subjects or target domains: population is its subject as well as its object. The best forms of governance are those which facilitate natural regulation (Gordon 1991: 18). Nowhere is this more apparent than in the case of the economy. Eighteenth-century thought had worked with the idea of 'oeconomy': that is, economy prefaced by 'oikos' (household), imbued with all the implications of 'possession, domestication and controlling action' which that entails (ibid.: 11). But Adam Smith gave voice to the idea that the laws and internal operations of economic activity were constituted by the free choices of economic agents.[1] Under these conditions, the art of governing involves knowing when not to act as well as when to act. Liberal governance thus emerges as a set of practices which recognises (and constantly re-recognises and rearticulates) its own limits. In the field of public welfare, for example, it continually problematises the relationship between public provision and economic growth and seeks to circumscribe its own interventions.

The same type of thinking applies to the governance of populations and individuals. From at least the nineteenth century on, population came to be understood as an entity with 'its own regularities, its own rate of deaths and diseases, its cycles of scarcity, etc.' (Foucault 1991: 101).[2] To govern a population is to govern in accordance with these regularities. Thus the provision of public relief should not be so high as to encourage procreation nor so low as to prevent it. Equally, the governance of individual subjects must promote 'natural' processes of self-regulation and provide the circumstances under which people may effectively govern themselves (Hindess 1996; Rose 1996a). For Dean (1992: 218) this is the linchpin of liberal governance. 'Liberal', he says, 'refers first of all to a form of practice of governance, one which sets itself against older hierocratic forms of rule, and attempts to specify some limits to that rule by means of appealing to a personal or private sphere.'

It is, however, only those whose responsibility and/or economic autonomy is already assumed who are to be governed at arm's length (cf. Garland 1997; Hindess 1996). Public welfare recipients, particularly the unemployed and sole parents, risk being positioned as subjects whose 'autonomy is . . . yet to be realised' (Hindess 1996: 73). In this position they are rendered subject to the 'individualising and responsibilising' technologies of professional, official and philanthropic interventions (Rose 1996a: 48–9). Their governance is thus underpinned by a range of disciplinary measures which, in their turn, are related to 'sovereign' considerations and the force of interdictory law.

The second main characteristic of liberal governance is that it is a calculated form of regulation. Liberal strategies tie government to the 'positive knowledge of human conduct' with the result that official activities 'become connected up to all manner of facts . . . techniques . . . and knowledgeable persons' (Rose 1996a: 44–5). Governmental decisions and actions need to be accountable and accounted for, justified in terms of their rationale and anticipated outcomes. The current and projected number of retired persons and the associated costs of national superannuation and pension programmes are thus based on a multiplicity of demographic, social and economic calculations.

Third, liberal governance utilises the 'apparatuses of security' – or insurantial technologies – as its major technology (Foucault 1991: 102). These insurantial technologies operate at a distance from their subjects and partially replace the older disciplinary technologies. They assume a free subject and operate to involve that subject in ensuring his or her own security. Public and private income security schemes (superannuation, sickness and unemployment benefits, child-care benefits, etc.) are one of their major components.

Rationalities, programmes and technologies of government

In tracing changes in governmental thought and action, it is useful to note Rose and Miller's (1992) distinction between political rationalities, programmes and technologies.

Political rationalities are ways of thinking about the dimensions and practices of governance: how government should operate; the ideals and principles to which it should be directed; the relationship between authorities and their subjects (Rose and Miller 1992: 178–9). As Gordon (1991: 2) puts it:

> A rationality of government will thus mean a way of thinking about the nature and practice of government (who can govern; what governing is; what or who is governed) capable of making some form of that activity thinkable and practicable to both its practitioners and those on whom it is practised.

As far as public welfare is concerned, political rationalities include all those forms of thought which consider the principles guiding the allocation of public funds and the grounds on which government intervention should rest. They entail questions of 'who should govern' (priests, philanthropists, employers or bureaucrats, for example), of 'what governing is' (reforming or disciplining the individual, providing public work and/or assistance in money or kind) and of 'what should be governed' (the poor themselves, a category called 'poverty', income distribution or labour force opportunities).

Programmes of government translate political rationalities into actual measures for governing populations: they involve theories, explanations and particular ways of both thinking and doing things (Rose and Miller 1992: 181–2). Thus, for example, social security programmes incorporate certain theories about the level of income needed to safeguard against unjustifiable hardship, suppositions about the relationships between equity, redistribution and competition, and notions about work incentive and benefit levels. These suppositions have practical effects: they produce particular levels of income support, determine who is and who is not eligible and shape administrative practices.

Finally, technologies of government represent the strategies, techniques and procedures used to put rationalities and their associated programmes into effect. Often dismissed as trivial in mainstream sociological accounts, these 'humble and mundane mechanisms' are important for governmentality theorists (Rose and Miller 1992: 183). For it is through them, through 'techniques of notation, computation and calculation, procedures of examination and assessment' that 'authorities seek to instantiate government' (ibid.). The technologies associated with public welfare include poverty line measurements to determine benefit levels, income and means testing to assess eligibility, and demographic and other statistical surveys to calculate and predict expenditure levels.

The rationalities, programmes and technologies of government are various and inconsistent. Despite this, it is possible to sketch broad patterns of change. The work of a number of commentators (Burchell 1991; Dean 1991, 1992; Gordon 1991; Lewi and Wickham 1996; O'Malley and Palmer 1996; Rose 1993, 1996a), suggests three major shifts in liberal governance over the past two centuries. Each of these shifts embodies a different political rationality concerning the relationship between the 'economic' and the 'social'. These changing rationalities shape the way in which dependent and independent populations are constituted as subjects of governance and give rise to corresponding changes in the programmes and technologies of governance surrounding public welfare.

In the following discussion, I follow the work of Gordon (1991) and Rose (1996a), in particular, although my way of labelling each major change is slightly different from theirs.

Managing the relations between dependent and independent populations: an overview

Classical liberal governance

To recap: classical liberal governance emerged in the nineteenth century as a critique of the eighteenth-century idea that there was an 'oeconomy' which could be known and directed along the lines of household management. Under the influence of classical economic thought, the economy – and the self-regulating activities of self-interested subjects – were marked off as objects outside the domain of direct governance. This belief combined with Malthusian ideas about the 'natural' laws governing population to give rise to a distinctive political rationality. The social fortunes of the nation were seen to hinge on its economic advancement, and economic advancement, in its turn, was seen to be dependent on governmental distance. The governmental task became one of securing the conditions under which the liberty/security of populations and individuals could expand and prosper.

In the field of public welfare this political rationality had well-known consequences, giving rise to its own characteristic set of programmes and technologies. During the eighteenth century the management of the poor in England had relied on the administrative apparatus established by the 1601 Poor Law. The local parish served as the unit of administration with funds provided out of compulsory rates which were locally assessed and collected. Wherever possible, the able-bodied were to work for their relief. The 'workhouse test', designed to prevent abuse, meant that in order to claim relief the indigent had to be prepared to enter the workhouse where they obtained indoor relief. However, workhouses came to be seen as expensive, inefficient and inhumane. In 1782 Gilbert's Act excluded the able-bodied from indoor relief and restricted it to the aged and disabled.

In 1834 the Poor Law Amendment Act was passed, marking a significant landmark in liberal governance. The Commission of Inquiry condemned outdoor relief in lieu of wages and proposed to make the workhouse test a reality. The principle of 'less eligibility' was given formal status: the person in receipt of relief was to receive it on terms which ensured that his/her condition was less eligible (less favourable) than the poorest independent labourer.[3] The new system also imposed a central board of national commissioners which oversaw the work of the parishes. It was heralded as a historic advance in the science of public administration because of its promise to introduce national uniformity and regulate the administration of relief.

Dean (1991, 1992) depicts the earlier seventeenth- and eighteenth-century modes of regulation as 'police of the poor'. This form of regulation involved a number of technologies whereby the poor were known, categorised and classified. The 'police of the poor' was a direct and interventionist form of administration. Here and elsewhere, the science of police 'dreamed of a time in which . . . the conduct of all persons . . . was to be specified and scrutinised in minute particulars, through detailed regulation of habitation, dress, manners and the like' (Rose 1996a: 43). It is worth noting, though, that the desire to link the poor to national goals through industry meant that the poor 'could never be abandoned to the vagaries of the labour-market' (Dean, 1992: 228). It was, in this sense at least, a kinder rationality than the one which currently shapes the dimensions of public welfare.

It is in comparison with these aspirations and practices that Dean suggests that the Poor Law Amendment Act signified a 'liberal break' in methods of management. The Amendment Act set 'definite limits' to the responsibilities of the state through excluding able-bodied men from relief and offering relief to their dependants only within the 'deterrent, less-eligible, institution of the workhouse' (ibid.: 232). Malthusian ideas concerning population growth and notions of a 'natural' scarcity, heralded by classical political economy, were significant factors in these developments (Dean 1991, 1992). Under these circumstances, emphasis shifted from the governance of individual persons – the poor – to governance of a category – poverty – and from direct to indirect forms of regulation.

It would be a mistake to overemphasise the 'liberal' nature of these changes. As we have seen, liberal governance incorporates, even depends on, illiberal elements. Rose (1996a) argues that both Foucault's 'disciplines of the body' and his 'biopolitics of the population' found their way into the programmes and technologies of classical liberal governance.[4] The disciplinary institutions – schools, prisons and workhouses – sought to produce the 'subjective conditions, the forms of self mastery, self regulation and self control, necessary to govern a nation now made up of free and "civilised" citizens' (ibid.: 44). At the same time, biopolitical strategies with their detailed inquiries and statistical calculations 'rendered intelligible the domains whose laws liberal government must know and respect' (ibid.).

A related but different point is made by Dean (1992), who contrasts the 'hyper-administrative' zeal of Benthamism with the 'anti-administrative, abolitionist' ideas characteristic of Malthusian thinking. He suggests that in the end it was the 'unique assemblage of Benthamism and Malthusianism' which finally characterised poor-law reform (Dean 1992: 241). Benthamism represented 'the triumph of the centralised, professional forms of administration of relief and welfare over localism, parochialism, . . . particularity, dispersion and even abolition', while Malthusianism sets both the 'ethical ideal' of the new economic form of governance and the limits to it through the category of the 'independent labourer, the self-responsible male breadwinner with his natural dependents' (ibid.). This uneasy coexistence of centralised intervention and individualised responsibility has continued to characterise the broad patterns of welfare provision from that time on.

Expansive liberal governance

By the late eighteenth century, poverty, unemployment and the health of the population were producing conflicts over the role of the state (Gordon 1991). Critics argued that the formulations of classical liberal governance had failed and there developed a formula of rule which 'lay somewhere between classical liberalism and nascent socialism' (Rose 1996a: 48). Under this formula, 'the state was to take responsibility for an array of technologies of government that would "social-ize" both individual citizenship and economic life in the name of collective security' (ibid.). While the market's autonomy was infringed, its security was to be protected through regulating the social infrastructure which made possible the conditions guaranteeing production and exchange (ibid.). The task of government thus became one of placing both 'economy' and 'citizen' within a 'social' context and developing programmes and technologies directed towards the public good and social solidarity.

The adoption of social insurance programmes in a number of northern European countries was one of the most significant examples of an expanded social domain subject to administrative and professional action. Bismarck's innovations in this field, with their explicit aim of containing the disaffection of the working classes, were among the first and best known of these measures. In Britain, the failure of the Poor Law to meet the changing conditions of an industrial society, the development of alternative systems of relief such as the Friendly Societies and the presence of newer notions of social administration produced the 1905 Inquiry. Both the Majority and the Minority Reports (see Royal Commission on the Poor Laws 1909) recommended the elimination of the current system of workhouses and relief administered by guardians. But the Minority Report, which was to become the more influential document, proposed that the whole system of poor relief be abandoned and replaced by social insurance. Following the directions advocated by the Minority Report, aged pensions were introduced in 1908 and insurance against sickness and unemployment in 1911.

Under social insurance, compulsory contributions for such things as old-age, unemployment and sickness benefits are paid by individuals and the benefits are distributed by the state. These measures constitute the moral and practical technologies whereby market/ self-help rationalities ('people should take care of their own futures') are combined with an acceptance of state direction ('the government will ensure that they do so'). More generally, social insurance schemes are part of the 'insurantial technologies' which Foucault (1979) nominated as the principal instruments of governmentality. They provide the means for 'the taming of chance' (Hacking 1990), for predicting and minimising the consequences of misfortune, and for encouraging or compelling citizens to act on their own behalf. They are a 'technology of government that shapes the life and security of the population, while also having implications at the level of the individual's comportment and self-discipline' (Garland 1997: 181).

Australia did not adopt social insurance programmes in its governance of public welfare. Instead, it instituted a 'social assistance' programme of income security which was thought to be better suited to the demographic profile and circumstances of the country. Under a social assistance programme, there is no system of compulsory insurance. Instead, benefits are paid to recipients on a means/income tested basis, with funds derived from national revenue. Using this as its basic form of assistance, Australia introduced aged and invalid pensions in 1908. This type of income-tested provision was followed in almost all of Australia's subsequent social security measures. (New Zealand adopted the same model.)

Critics argue that social assistance marginalises and individualises those dependent on it. Recipients, precisely because there has been no prior payment of contributions, are construed as dependent on public funds and a burden on the tax-payer. A hierarchy of desert and blame is established, with some (old-age pensioners, for example) seen to be more worthy than others (the unemployed and sole parents in particular). The differences between social assistance and social insurance should not be overemphasised, however. In actuality there has always been a 'solidaristic' element to the Australian social assistance programmes in that they embody a collective response to a range of economic exigencies. Equally, social insurance programmes have always embodied an individualising and marginalising dimension. They are invariably underpinned by a 'less-eligible' form of assistance for those who have been unable to pay contributions or whose claim to assistance has been exhausted. Further, social insurance remains, in essence, a form of *poor* relief. Higher income earners, if and when they rely on state benefits, are likely to have other forms of financial support. The 'class' character of social insurance leaves it open to the same kind of marginalising logic as that which affects social assistance, even if to a lesser degree.

To return to the historical picture. Following the introduction of income security measures in the early part of this century, western governments expanded their public welfare systems. The pattern and pace of this expansion differed. In Northern America and New Zealand the 1930s' depression provided a major spur to the development of national schemes of relief. North America was introduced to Roosevelt's New Deal and New Zealand to a number of programmes which expanded its earlier welfare measures. In other cases, it was the Second World War which heralded the second major set of welfare initiatives. In Britain, there was the Beveridge plan with its aspiration to end poverty and unemployment and its significant expansion of public housing, education, health and income assistance schemes.[5] The historical pattern was similar in Australia, where the Second World War saw the Commonwealth Government assume pre-emptive powers in income tax collections and greater powers in welfare legislation. As a result, the 1940s brought about the consolidation of child allowances, unemployment and sickness benefits, the widow's pension and public housing.

Developments such as these provided a collective response to the economic risks faced by individuals through their lifetimes. As a result of welfarism, new relations between the state and citizen were formed (Rose 1996a: 48). The subject as 'private individual' was no longer so distinct from the subject as 'public citizen' as closer associations were forged between public procedures and the fortunes of individuals in their private lives (ibid.). As part of this process, the connection between the 'economic' and the 'social' was redrawn. The two spheres emerged as more or less interdependent entities and governance was directed towards their joint optimisation (Rose 1996b: 338).

The postwar period also saw the expansion of Titmuss's 'occupational' and 'fiscal' welfare domains. Across western societies, middle to high income employees in both the private and the public sector benefited from the growth of superannuation, sickness and paid leave entitlements as well as from a range of allowances which could be claimed through the taxation system. These developments advantaged those in the primary labour market over casual, contract or part-time workers, and men over women. Their overall impact was regressive.[6]

Keynesian economics was a central component of the political rationalities underlying the growth of government activity. By outlining the conditions under which intervention could secure not only the welfare but also the prosperity of the nation, Keynesian thought encouraged liberal governance to expand the limits of its rule (Rose 1996a). Although this was challenged from the outset – most notably in Hayek's *Road to Serfdom* (1944) – the basic tenets of welfarism were largely sustained during the 1950s and 1960s. It was not until the 1970s, when, ironically, a number of countries were 'rediscovering' their poor and in some instances attempting to do something about it,[7] that welfarism came seriously under attack.

Advanced liberal governance

Commentators are agreed that from around the 1970s there was a sea change in western economies. The components and causes of this change are many and various. They include slowing economic growth rates, a tendency towards deindustrialisation in Europe and the United States, and the growth of long-term unemployment. More specifically, the collapse of the Bretton Woods agreement and the OPEC oil crisis produced long-lasting instability in all the major economies with effects experienced well into the early 1980s (Hirst and Thompson 1996). The domestic uncertainty caused by this and other factors encouraged financiers and manufacturers to seek new markets while national governments increasingly moved in the direction of market deregulation (ibid.).

The extent to which these changes in international financial and trading markets have produced a more open or 'global' economy where 'anything can be made anywhere on the face of the earth and sold anywhere else on the face of the earth' and in which 'national economies fade away' (Thurow 1996: 9) is arguable. It is, however, fair to conclude that a 'substantial disconnect' arises 'between global business firms with a world view and national governments that focus on the welfare of their voters' (ibid.). In this context, Hirst and Thompson (1995, 1996), despite their caution over the globalisation thesis, point to an internationalisation of economic relations which places limits on any national government's capacity to pursue policies which diverge significantly from the norms established by international financial markets.

These changes lie behind what Rose (1996b) calls the 'de-socialisation' of economic governance. The economy which was to be managed for social purposes under welfarism was a *national* economy which could be facilitated and understood along territorial lines. The internationalisation of economic relations means that an economy can no longer be seen as 'naturally coextensive with the realm of a nation-state' (ibid.: 338). Instead, 'theorists and practitioners alike now construe economic relations as "globalized" and this new spatialization of the economy is coupled with arguments that flexible economic relations need to be established in particular localities' (ibid.). As a result, 'the economic well-being of the nation and of its population can no longer be so easily mapped upon one another and governed according to principles of mutual maximisation' (ibid.). Under these conditions, governance of the national economy in the name of the social gives way to the government of particular spheres of economic interest (ibid.; see also Hindess 1998).

Another important development has been the shift, or partial shift, from standardised mass production (Fordism) to 'flexible specialisation' (post-Fordism). Fordism incorporated many of the programmes and technologies of expansive liberal governance. It relied on state intervention in the economy to ensure stabilised mass markets, accepted the need for the social wage and looked to the regulation of international markets (Castells 1991; Probert 1994: 102). According to Castells (1991: 135), it was 'less . . . a system of mass production, more . . . a total way of life'. This 'Fordist way of life' began to falter in the 1970s when it was confronted by falling productivity growth, international competition and sustained upward pressures on direct and social wages. It was replaced, or partially replaced, by an industrial rationality which emphasised flexibility, strategic choice, niche markets, multiskilling and enterprise bargaining.[8]

One of the most significant elements of these changes is the reduced capacity of the nation-state, particularly as far as its ability to deliver broadly based welfare programmes is concerned. Bob Jessop (1994: 253) suggests that post-Fordism has seen a shift from a 'welfare' to a 'workfare' state. This, he says, has been accompanied by 'a tendential "hollowing out" of the national state' in which the nation-state's capacities are 'reorganised on supranational, national, regional or local, and translocal levels' (ibid.).[9] As a result, western governments have been involved in a concerted attempt to reduce wage, salary and taxation levels and, above all, to restrict public expenditure (Pusey 1991). These efforts have been accompanied by a shift in political priorities and administrative style, leading to a downgrading of traditional social democratic concerns in favour of technocratic management and economic efficiency (Du Gay 1994; Halligan and Power 1992; Yeatman 1987, 1990).[10]

It is within this context that advanced liberalism progressively deploys the language of economic theory to manage social and political affairs. If the economy was a self-governing entity under classical political economy and an interdependent domain under Keynesian economics, it is now an inclusive mode of operation which subsumes the social (Muetzelfeldt 1992; Pusey 1991). Gordon (1991: 43) suggests that American neo-liberalism 'proposes a global redescription of the social as a form of the economic'. This operation, he says:

> works by a progressive enlargement of the territory of economic theory by a series of redefinitions of its object, starting out from the neo-classical formula that economics concerns the study of all behaviours involving the allocation of scarce resources to alternative ends. Now it is proposed that economics concerns all purposive conduct entailing strategic choices between alternative paths, means and instruments; or, yet more broadly, *all rational conduct* ... and finally, all conduct, rational or irrational, which responds to its environment in a non-random fashion, or 'recognises reality'.
>
> (Ibid. Emphasis in original)

In programmatic terms this means that the market is progressively applied to areas previously outside it. The market becomes 'both an ideal and an objective to be achieved' with technologies designed to 'locate people and groups within these fields so that they will act in ways that produce the outcomes policy makers intended' (Muetzelfeldt 1992: 174). Clients become customers, health and welfare services are made subject to purchaser–provider models, vouchers and other user-pays technologies are introduced. These strategies have been accompanied by a fragmentation of the 'social' into individual interests and smaller sectional groups based on personal interest (Rose 1996b).

All this has had significant consequences as far as the governance of public welfare is concerned. Over the past two decades there have been widespread attempts to reduce public expenditure on social security through increasing surveillance over beneficiaries, cutting and streamlining benefits, introducing and/or tightening income tests and invoking parental responsibility for young adults previously eligible for unemployment benefit or student allowances in their own right. These strategies have made the most serious inroads into benefits targeted at groups such as unemployed youth or single parents. They have, however, been less successful in cutting programmes with a more universal appeal or coverage. Partly because of this, governments have not been able to cut spending on income security by the desired amounts.

Proponents of New Right thinking argue that welfarism has undermined both economic processes and the coping capacities of individuals (e.g. Murray 1984; Tapper 1990). So where classical liberalism had seen the self-interested individual and the self-regulating market as existing, quasi-natural zones, advanced liberalism sees 'enterprise' – the enterprising society, the enterprising subject and enterprising economic endeavour – as things which it must actively work to *re*create (Gordon 1991). Its task, at least in part, is remedial: it must undo the damage of expansive liberalism and inculcate a political climate in which self-sufficiency is desired and learned.[11] People who have come to rely on welfare must learn to see dependence as 'less-eligible' in moral as well as economic terms. This is precisely the point behind the 'new welfare' policies of Britain and the United States. Even though they disassociate themselves from the economic policies of their immediate predecessors, both Tony Blair and Bill Clinton continue to deploy the same broad rationality. Their contention that the best form of welfare is that which provides people with the skills to do without it speaks to the heart of advanced liberal notions concerning active participation and the nature of citizenship.

The practical effects of the new economic rationalities are particularly evident in a range of programmes which aim to transform the unemployed person into a 'job-seeker' (Dean 1995; Walters 1994, 1996). As Dean (1995: 576) puts it, such programmes are concerned to 'render the individual an active entrepreneur of his or her own self, ready and able to take up such opportunities that the labour market, social provision, education, and social network may provide'. The drive to recreate a natural self-sufficiency has brought about new work tests, new income tests and new training schemes which aim to force or encourage people to take up work or, failing that, to depend on their family rather than the state. Taken together, such measures constitute a moral technology designed to produce a changed subjectivity among the current and potential beneficiaries of public welfare (Muetzelfeldt 1992).

Despite the emphasis on self-actualisation, the strategies aimed at the unemployed are often direct and disciplinary. As a suspect population, the unemployed are subject to specific requirements that they attend interviews, apply for a specified number of jobs over a nominated period and maintain records of their activities. Documents such as the 'job-seeker's diary' must be produced at regular intervals and can be inspected at any time. 'Work for the dole' schemes are prime examples of disciplinary programmes which at the same time speak to the desire to create an 'enterprising' culture which eschews dependency. They need to be understood in this context rather than as a modern variant of older outdoor relief programmes which had, at their heart, the attempt to provide relief in particular economic circumstances.

In the current economic and political climate private forms of insurance are prospering. A 'new prudentialism' arises in which insurance against eventualities such as unemployment, ill-health and old age becomes a private choice rather than a communal responsibility, with the insured person construed as a rational and autonomous agent (O'Malley 1996). Consequently, 'social in-surance as a principle of social solidarity, gives way to a kind of privatisation of risk management' (Rose 1996a: 58). In effect, this means that the state progressively disengages from providing, guaranteeing and/or monitoring insurance schemes, leaving the individual 'free' to make his or her own choices.

Advanced liberal rationalities have also affected occupational and fiscal welfare programmes. While these are more attuned to the language of self-actualisation than are public welfare programmes, many occupational benefits have been negotiated through unions or professional associations (thus, for example, superannuation, sickness leave and maternity benefit). This runs counter to the in-dividualised ethos of advanced liberalism. For this reason, collective benefits have become increasingly subject to enterprise bargaining and/or individual productivity agreements. Under these conditions, the regressive elements of these schemes, and their tendency to favour men over women, is greatly amplified.

The net effect of these changes is an intensification of practices which classify and divide people. This has significant implica-tions for the ways in which citizenship is currently constituted and experienced.

Critique: fragmented citizenship

A number of theorists (e.g. Cruikshank 1996; Dean 1995; Miller and Rose 1988, 1990; Pixley 1993; Rose 1992, 1996b) have maintained that there has been a significant shift in the nature of the participatory bonds which constitute and join people as common members of a shared sociopolitical order. Miller and Rose (1988: 24) speak of 'an apparently decisive displacement of the political rationalities which construed citizenship in terms of solidarity, contentment, welfare and a sense of security' towards the principles of self-help and individual enterprise. Subjects are now to be joined by contractual and market relations, and positioned as common members of an exchange economy (O'Malley 1996). This construction of the normative subject sets the gainfully employed against the jobless, rich against poor, and men against women. The prototype subject of advanced liberalism has secure employment prospects, a chance to experiment, and time to work on him (*sic*) self. This masculinisation of political discourse means that a moral lacuna occurs when it comes to reciprocity, care of others and collective effort.

This shift has led Rose (1996a, 1996b) and others to speak of the 'death' or 'reconfiguration' of the social domain created by welfarist forms of governance. At least three things are suggested here. First, and as we have just seen, it is proposed that contractual relations have come to substitute for the common bonds of reciprocity and mutuality which shaped social citizenship in the earlier part of the twentieth century. Second, it is argued that under advanced liberalism 'strategies of pluralisation and autonomisation' fragment the broad plane of the social created by welfare technologies (Rose 1996a: 56). In its place arise smaller, individualised spaces of personal responsibility: 'micro-moral domains' built on sectional communities (ibid.: 57). Third, there is said to be a reversal of the processes whereby the state became involved in governance and was itself subject to governance. Advanced liberalism embodies a wish for 'a kind of "de-governmentalisation of the state" and "de-statization of government" – a phenomenon which is linked to amputation of the notion of the social' (ibid.: 56).

Each of these factors has a direct bearing on the relationship between public welfare and citizenship and on the capacity of welfare recipients to meet the criteria of full and active citizenship. The subordination of mutuality to contractual relations is reproduced in the subordination of welfare to market. The effect is to remove, or partially remove, the 'social' elements of T.H. Marshall's three-fold classification of citizenship. As a result, the infrastructure of state benefits which allows people to participate in the public and political life of their society is endangered and eligibility for citizenship is narrowed and rendered less equal. Next, the 'fragmentation of the social' runs directly counter to Beveridge's (1942: 6) aspirations for a *comprehensive* policy of social progress' directed against 'Want, Disease, Ignorance, Squalor and Idleness' (my emphasis). It also intensifies the dividing practices whereby some subjects – and in our context, those dependent on public welfare – are judged to be deficient and excluded from full citizenship. Finally, the 'de-governmentalisation of the state' means that governments are less likely to be held responsible for managing the income security of their populations while the 'de-statization of government' means income security is less likely to become the province of the state.

The crux of the matter is that advanced liberal rationality reduces citizenship to a notion of productive effort based on paid work. Under these circumstances, older notions that citizenship is expressed through participation in civic or public life is effectively sized down to the idea that citizenship can only be realised through paid work and/or financial investment. This produces a discourse which can neither recognise nor articulate the economic, social and political contributions of those dependent on public welfare. It also strengthens the longstanding tradition by which the domestic and voluntary work generally undertaken by women is rendered invisible. Economic productivity, narrowly defined, becomes the hallmark of the independent and enterprising subject. The marginalising and divisive effects of this discourse are greatly amplified by the tendency to 'respond to the sufferer as though they were the author of their own misfortunes' (Rose 1996a: 59). Enjoining independence and enterprise when jobs are scarce both blames victims and aims to reform them for non-existent possibilities.

But it is important to acknowledge that these trends are not new (Rose, 1996b). Part of the point of this chapter has been to argue that public welfare has always been problematic because it involves public payments for people considered dependent. The way in which this difficulty has been mediated has repeatedly posed questions concerning the balance between intervention and non-intervention. Public welfare clients have consistently been subject to the normalising discourses of social work and to the more direct and disciplinary forms of state intervention. And from the Poor Law on, the administration of relief has invariably involved judgement, classification and division. The proposals of Bentham and the Webbs, for example, stand as testimony to that (Dean 1992; Rose 1996b). The contribution of advanced liberalism is not to invent those practices but to refurbish them, giving them new life and meaning, after the temporary relaxation offered by the rationalities of welfarism and social citizenship.

Tensions and the pressure for change

Placing current developments within a broader historical context shows that contemporary rationalities are just one of a number of possible responses to a longer-standing issue. This robs advanced liberalism of any claim to be a fixed, necessary or natural way of going about things. History records that political rationalities have changed over time and are likely to do so again. There is, then, no reason to believe that we are destined to travel down an increasingly economically rational path. Instead, there are good grounds for believing that we may *not* do so. Despite the elegance of economic rationality, the current system is characterised by tensions and points of conflict which make it unlikely that the market will be an unqualified victor in the foreseeable future. These tensions or, to borrow Dorothy Smith's (1974, 1979) phrase, 'lines of fault' operate at both a micro and a macro level. They set the scene for programmatic change and ultimately, perhaps, for a more general shift in governing rationalities.

At a micro level there are manifold fissures which help to disrupt the smooth flowing of organisational design.[12] Opposition is expressed by unemployed people when they recognise that labour scarcity rather than their own lack of skills has produced their jobless state and/or when they struggle to stay on benefits rather than take jobs which evidently do not suit them. In 'coming up against the system', recipients may decide to observe only the formalities of the job-seeking requirements imposed upon them. Their attempts to circumvent the rules may be assisted by officials who have long-standing allegiances to different rationalities or have come to recognise the implausibilities of advanced liberalism. Under these circumstances, checks on beneficiaries may be performed in a less systematic way than officially required and gaps and inconsistencies in job-seeking diaries wholly or partially ignored.

At a macro level a major tension is exhibited in the continuing shortfall between the demands placed on the public welfare system and the resources available to it. Resources for the distribution and administration of national income security schemes have either fallen in absolute terms or failed to keep pace with the increase in demand caused by rising unemployment levels and demographic change. The governmental response, as we have seen, has been to cut benefits wherever possible and to promote an ethos of enterprise which marginalises the welfare endeavour. Governments have also introduced computerised technologies which assist in information collection and client surveillance while reducing the numbers of staff employed to administer social security schemes. These strategies, however, have not succeeded in eradicating the shortfall between demand and resources. The increased burden born by charitable services as well as continued talk of the 'new poor' and of a growing 'under class' are testimony to that.

Such developments – and the marketisation of welfare more generally – generate contestation. Civil rights proponents worry about computerised surveillance; welfare lobbyists argue that benefit levels should be sufficient to allow people to participate in their community; union officials draw attention to the erosion of wages and job conditions; social commentators predict that rising levels of income inequality are producing an 'under class' of impoverished minorities. Each of these concerns appeals to wider values: democratic rights, participation, economic equality and social stability. Taken together, they provide the base for a critique of advanced liberalism and for the formulation of alternative political rationalities which recognise mutuality and different forms of political and economic association (see, for example, European Commission 1994; Hirst 1994; Hutton 1995.)[13]

Conflicting rationalities and political critiques open up spaces to imagine that things might be different. Such imaginings cannot lend themselves to a final point, an end claim about the nature of social justice. Poststructural theory, in positing the discursive and historical nature of all justice claims, cannot provide universal notions of the good society. What it can do is create the conditions under which new claims can be heard and registered (cf. Fraser 1981; Phillips 1993; Yeatman 1994). In line with this, the poststructural vision of a better society must recognise the heterogeneous and multifaceted nature of any justice agenda (Phillips 1993; Hirst 1994; Fraser 1997). This does not, however, necessarily involve abandoning the older notions of justice associated with socialism. The task, as Nancy Fraser (1997) argues, is to combine parts of the socialist agenda with newer claims relating to the diversity of cultural claims and interests.

Fraser's arguments reaffirm the need to provide an adequate income for all. If political and social difference and the multiplicity of justice claims are to recognised, then we must have an economic base from which people can variously voice and practise their own versions of political and economic participation. This leads, more or less directly, to the notion of a guaranteed minimum income (GMI) or CI (citizens' income). But it needs to be remembered that such proposals have gained support in the ranks of the Right as well as the Left. As part of the advanced liberal reform agenda, they are used to justify user-pays measures, vouchers and the reduction of direct service provision. Any alternative case for a guaranteed income therefore needs to be made in conjunction with a broader set of proposals which enhance social solidarity, mutuality and associative democracy. Only then would a guaranteed income have the potential to assist in the formulation of different versions of democratic practice. The payment, as Tony Fitzpatrick (1996: 314) argues, needs to be of a 'social dividend' nature and sufficiently high as to untie the reliance on earnings-related sources of income.

Finally, the analysis developed in this chapter suggests that income support should be provided without a requirement for people to identify themselves as particular sorts of claimants – unemployed, sole parent, widow, aged, etc. – as it is the dividing practices associated with this kind of administration which marginalises recipients and enforces particular forms of incorporation into designated subject groups (Foucault 1988). By the same token it is important to argue for the dissolution of the work/welfare nexus which has consistently produced a myriad of classifications, categories and judgements surrounding eligibility and less eligibility. What we need instead is a political language which recognises the necessarily interdependent and interactive relations between subjects. This could provide one avenue for disrupting advanced liberalism and, with it, some of the longer punitive traditions behind the governance of public welfare.

Notes

1 Although placing limits on the capacities of governments to regulate economic activity, Adam Smith did not explicitly propose an 'economic' domain which was separate from a 'moral' or 'social' sphere (Rose 1994: 46). For Adam Smith, 'political economy was a moral science' (ibid.). The idea of the economy as a separate domain, although perhaps implicit in Adam Smith's thinking (Hindess 1998), was in fact a later product of nineteenth-century classical political economy. In its turn, this conception of the economy was 'a key condition for the separation out of a social domain' (Rose 1996b: 337). 'Society' can be seen as an 'invention of the social scientists of the nineteenth century': the 'sum of the bonds and relations which is governed by its own laws' (Rose 1994: 46). (Note that both 'economy' and 'society' were envisaged as *national* spheres, largely commensurate with territorial boundaries. This was to be challenged by the globalisation of economic relations in the latter part of the twentieth century, (which is discussed later in this chapter).

2 Foucault (1991: 101) suggests that prior to the emergence of population 'it was impossible to conceive of the art of government except on the model of the family'; whereas, 'from the moment when, on the contrary, population appears absolutely irreducible to the family, the latter becomes of secondary importance compared to population, . . . no longer, that is to say, a model, but a segment' (ibid.). Under these circumstances, control becomes indirect and circumspect, and previous familial models of governance, with all the suppositions of. direct control and detailed knowledge which they entail, are rendered obsolete or at least partially so.

3 This ruling subsequently turned out to be virtually impossible to administer in the face of large-scale unemployment in the manufacturing towns and outdoor relief was sanctioned in a number of places.

4 Foucault (1979) distinguished the 'power over life' ('bio-power') from the 'power to take life'. He associated the 'power to take life' with the pre-modern sovereign state and the 'power over life' ('bio-power') with modern and early modern forms of governance. He argued that, approximately from the seventeenth century, 'bio-power' emerged in two basic forms, constituting:

> two poles of development linked together by a whole intermediary of relations. One of these poles, the first to be formed it seems . . . centred on the body as a machine . . . ensured by the procedures of power characterised by the *disciplines; an anatamo-politics of the human body*. The second, formed somewhat later, focused on the species body, the body imbued with the mechanics of life . . . [its] supervision was effected through an

entire series of interventions and *regulatory controls: a bio-politics of the population.*

> (Foucault 1979: 139; emphasis in original)

In both its forms, 'bio-power' places individuals and populations as the *object* of governance. In this sense, it constitutes one side of the 'object/subject' tension with which contemporary liberal governance constantly juggles.

5 The depression had seen the introduction of the Unemployment Assistance Board (1935) which paid relief to those whose contributions had run out.

6 Compared with the highly visible, quantified characteristics of public programmes, expenditure on occupational and fiscal welfare remained a relatively unquantified and unknown quantity. The schemes were truly seen as something earned: a right, a payment, a justifiable claim. Their impact was regressive as they sustained or exacerbated existing patterns of privilege and exclusion. They also helped to occlude the fact that earlier welfare initiatives and economic growth had not eradicated poverty.

7 For Australia, the Commission of Inquiry into Poverty (1975) and the Whitlam Government's initiatives in the fields of health, education and welfare are critical developments of this kind.

8 The extent and causes of these changes are open to dispute. Proponents of the flexible-specialisation school (e.g. Piore and Sabel 1984) are opposed by regulation theorists and neo-Marxian analyses (e.g. Aglietta 1987). For a useful overview of these disputes, see Amin 1994 or Clegg 1991.

9 There has, however, been considerable variation in national response to the changes outlined here. Some nations have adopted a 'post-Fordist' approach incorporating certain flexible, democratic practices; others a so-called 'neo-Fordist' direction which relies on the achievement of market efficiencies (see Brown 1996). In determining which, or what combination, of these approaches will be followed much seems to depend on the previous institutional and political relationships between labour and capital (Gottfried 1995).

10 These developments exacerbated already existing tendencies towards increasing income inequality and rising levels of unemployment. Poverty continued to increase throughout the 1970s and 1980s, the burden being increasingly borne by women and households with dependants (Cass 1985; Harris 1989).

11 In this context, Barbara Cruikshank, in her analysis of the Californian Task Force to Promote Self Esteem and Personal and Social Responsibility, brings our attention to the self-esteem projects of welfare professionals. She suggests that self-esteem is 'a technology . . . for evaluating and acting upon ourselves so that the police, the

guards and the doctors do not have to' (Cruikshank 1996: 234). She points out that citizens who achieve self-esteem or 'revolution from within' are citizens 'doing the right thing; they join programs, volunteer, but most importantly, work on and improve their self image . . . at all times, self-esteem calls on individuals to act, to participate' (ibid.).

12 As far as I know no systematic study of these points of internal resistance has been done and it would be hard to imagine the political and methodological conditions under which such a study could be safely undertaken. My comments therefore rely on conversations with people receiving social security benefits and on the accounts of colleagues in the public sector.

13 Public welfare has proved more vulnerable to the market rationalities than have either health or education. The historic idea that income is normally earned – or should wherever possible be earned – through the market, stands as a 'truth' which makes it more difficult to mount a sustained popular argument against welfare cuts (particularly when such cuts have been couched in terms of promoting self-sufficiency) than against the loss of hospital beds or primary schools.

References

Aglietta, M. (1987) *A Theory of Capitalist Regulation: The US Experience*, London: Verso.

Amin, A. (1994) 'Post-Fordism: models, fantasies and strategies of transition', in A. Amin (ed.), *Post-Fordism: A Reader*, Oxford: Basil Blackwell.

Barry, A., Osborne, T. and Rose, N. (1993) 'Liberalism, neo-liberalism and governmentality: an introduction' *Economy and Society*, 22, 3: 265–6

Best, S. and Kellner, D. (1991) *Postmodern Theory, Critical Interrogations*, London: Macmillan.

Beveridge, W. (1942) *Social Insurance and Allied Services* (Cmd 6404), London: HMSO.

Brown, P. (1996) 'Education, globalisation and economic development', *Journal of Education Policy*, 11, 1: 1–25.

Bryson, L. (1992) *Welfare and the State: Who Benefits?*, London: Macmillan.

Burchell, G. (1991) 'Peculiar interests: civil society and governing "the system of natural liberty"' in G. Burchell, C. Gordon and P. Miller (eds), *The Foucault Effect: Studies in Governmentality*, Chicago: University of Chicago Press.

Cass, B. (1985) 'The changing face of poverty in Australia 1972–1982', *Australian Feminist Studies*, no 1, Summer: 67–9.

Castells, M. (1991) *The Informational City*, Oxford: Basil Blackwell.

Clegg, S.R. (1991) *Modern Organisations: Organisation Studies in the Postmodern World*, London: Sage, Lonio.

Corrigan, P. and Leonard, P. (1978) *Social Work Practice Under Capitalism: A Marxist Approach*, London: Macmillan.

Cruikshank, B. (1996) 'Revolutions within: self-government and self-esteem', in A. Barry, T. Osborne and N. Rose (eds), *Foucault and Political Reason*, London, UCL Press (first published in *Economy and Society*, 22, 3 (1993): 327– 43).

Dean, M. (1991) *The Constitution of Poverty: Toward a Genealogy of Liberal Governance*, London: Routledge.

Dean, M. (1992) 'A genealogy of the government of poverty', *Economy and Society*, 21, 3: 215–52.

Dean, M. (1995) 'Governing the unemployed in an active society', *Economy and Society*, 24, 4: 559–83.

Du Gay, P. (1994) 'Making up managers: bureaucracy, enterprise and the liberal art of separation', *British Journal of Sociology*, 45, 4: 655–74.

European Commission (1994) *European Social Policy: A Way Forward for the Union. A White Paper*, Luxembourg: Office for Official Publications of the European Commission.

Fitzpatrick, T. (1996) 'Postmodernism, welfare and radical politics', *Journal of Social Policy*, 25, 3: 303–20.

Foucault, M. (1979) *The History of Sexuality*, Harmondsworth, Middx.: Penguin.

Foucault, M. (1982) 'The subject and power', in H.L. Dreyfus and P. Rabinow, *Foucault: Beyond Structuralism and Hermeneutics*, Brighton, Sussex: Harvester Press.

Foucault, M. (1988) 'Social security', in L. D. Kritzman (ed.), *Politics, Philosophy and Culture Interviews and Other Writings*, New York: Routledge.

Foucault, M. (1991) 'Governmentality', in G. Burchell, C. Gordon, and P. Miller (eds), *The Foucault Effect: Studies in Governmentality*, Chicago: University of Chicago Press.

Fraser, N. (1981) 'Foucault on modern power: empirical insights and normative confusions', *Praxis International*, 1, 3: 72–7.

Fraser, N. (1997) *Justice Interruptus: Critical Reflections on the "Postsocialist" Condition*, New York: Routledge.

Galper, J. (1980) *Social Work Practice: A Radical Perspective*, Englewood Cliffs, NJ: Prentice-Hall.

Garland, D. (1997) '"Governmentality" and the problem of crime', *Theoretical Criminology*, 1, 2: 173–214.

Gordon, C. (1991) 'Governmental rationality: an introduction', in G. Burchell, C. Gordon and P. Miller (eds), *The Foucault Effect: Studies in Governmentality*, Chicago: University of Chicago Press.

Gottfried, H. (1995) 'Developing neo-Fordism: a comparative perspective', *Critical Sociology*, 21, 3: 49–70.

Gough, I. (1979) *The Political Economy of the Welfare State*, London: Macmillan.

Hacking, I. (1990) *The Taming of Chance*, Cambridge: Cambridge University Press.

Halligan, J. and Power, J. (1992) *Political Management in the 1990s*, Oxford: Oxford University Press.

Harris, P. (1989) *Child Poverty, Inequality and Social Justice*, Child Poverty Policy Review no. 1, Melbourne: Brotherhood of St Laurence.

Hayek, F. von (1944) *The Road to Serfdom*, London: Routledge and Kegan Paul.

Hindess, B. (1996) 'Liberalism, socialism and democracy: variations on a governmental theme', in A. Barry, T. Osborne and N. Rose (eds), *Foucault and Political Reason*, London: UCL Press.

Hindess, B. (1998) 'Neoliberalism and the national economy', in M. Dean and B. Hindess (eds), *Governing Australia: Studies in Contemporary Rationalities of Government*, Cambridge: Cambridge University Press.

Hirst, P. (1994) *Associative Democracy: New Forms of Economic and Social Governance*, Cambridge: Polity Press.

Hirst, P. and Thompson, G. (1995). 'Globalisation and the future of the nation-state', *Economy and Society*, 24, 3: 409–42.

Hirst, P. and Thompson, G. (1996) *Globalisation in Question: The International Economy and the Possibilities of Governance*, London: Pluto Press.

Hutton, W. (1995) *The State We're In*, London: Cape.

Jessop, B. (1994) 'Post-Fordism and the State', in A. Amin (ed.), *Post-Fordism: A Reader*, Oxford: Basil Blackwell.

Jones, C. (1983) *State Social Work and the Working Class*, London: Macmillan.

Lewi, H. and Wickham, G. (1996) 'Modern urban government: a Foucaultian perspective', *Urban Policy and Research*, 14, 1: 51–64.

Miller, P. and Rose, N. (1988) 'Political rationalities and technologies of government', paper presented at Colloquium on Language and Politics, University of Helsinki, subsequently published in *Politikka*, 1989, in Finnish translation.

Miller P. and Rose, N. (1990). 'Governing economic life', *Economy and Society*, 19, 1: 1–31.

Muetzelfeldt, M. (1992) 'Economic rationalism in its social context', in M. Muetzelfeldt (ed.), *State, Society and Politics in Australia*, Melbourne: Pluto Press.

Murray, C. (1984) *Losing Ground: American Social Policy, 1950–1980*, New York: Basic Books.

O'Malley, P. (1996) 'Risk and responsibility', in A. Barry, T. Osborne and N. Rose (eds), *Foucault and Political Reason*, London: UCL Press.

O'Malley, P. and Palmer, D. (1996) 'Post-Keynesian policing', *Economy and Society*, 25, 2: 137–55.

O'Malley, P., Weir, R. and Shearing, C. (1997) 'Governmentality, criticism and politics', *Economy and Society*, 26, 4: 501–17.

Phillips, A. (1993) *Democracy and Difference*, Cambridge: Polity Press.

Piore, M. and Sabel, C. (1984) *The Second Industrial Divide: Possibilities for Prosperity*, New York: Basic Books.

Pixley, J. (1993) *Citizenship and Employment: Investigating Post-industrial Options*, Cambridge: Cambridge University Press.

Probert, B. (1994) 'Globalisation, economic restructuring and the state', in S. Bell and B. Head (eds), *State, Economy and Public Policy in Australia*, Melbourne: Oxford University Press.

Pusey, M. (1991) *Economic Rationalism in Canberra: A Nation Building State Changes its Mind*, Melbourne: Cambridge University Press.

Rose, N. (1992) 'Governing the enterprising self', in P. Heelas and M. Morris (eds), *The Values of the Enterprise Culture: The Moral Debate*, London: Unwin Hyman.

Rose, N. (1993) 'Government, authority and expertise in advanced liberalism', *Economy and Society*, 22, 3: 283–327.

Rose, N. (1994) 'Regulating the social', in M. Valverde (ed.), *Radically Re-thinking Regulation*, Workshop Report, Toronto: Centre of Criminology, University of Toronto, 46–49.

Rose, N. (1996a) 'Governing "advanced" liberal democracies', in A. Barry, T. Osborne and N. Rose (eds), *Foucault and Political Reason*, London: UCL Press.

Rose, N. (1996b) 'The death of the social', *Economy and Society*, 25, 3: 327–56.

Rose, N. and Miller, P. (1992) 'Political power beyond the state: problematics of government', *British Journal of Sociology*, 43, 2: 173–205.

Royal Commission on the Poor Laws and Relief of Distress (1909) *Report*, Cd 4499, London: HMSO [Majority Report]; *Separate Report* by the Reverend Prebendary H. Russell Wakefield, Mr Francis Chandler and Mrs Sydney Webb [Minority Report].

Smart, B. (1986) 'The politics of truth and the problem of hegemony', in D. Couzens Hoy (ed.), *Foucault: A Critical Reader*, Oxford: Basil Blackwell.

Smith, D. (1974) 'The social construction of documentary reality', *Sociological Inquiry*, 44, 4: 257–68.

Smith, D. (1979) 'A sociology for women', in A. Sherman and E. Torton Beck (eds), *The Prism of Sex: Essays in the Sociology of Women*, Madison: University of Wisconsin Press.

Tapper, A. (1990) *The Family in the Welfare State*, North Sydney: Allen and Unwin and the Australian Institute for Public Policy.

Thurow, L. (1996) *The Future of Capitalism: How Today's Economic Forces Will Shape Tomorrow's World*, London: Allen and Unwin.

Titmuss, R.M. (1963) *Essays on the Welfare State*, 2nd edn, London: George Allen and Unwin.

Walters, W. (1994) 'The discovery of unemployment: new forms for the government of poverty', *Economy and Society*, 23, 3: 265–90.

Walters, W. (1996) 'The demise of unemployment', *Politics and Society*, 24, 3: 197–219.

Wearing, M. and Berreen, R. (1994) *Welfare and Social Policy in Australia: The Distribution of Advantage*, Sydney: Harcourt Press.

Wilson, E. (1997) *Women and the Welfare State*, London: Tavistock.

Yeatman, A. (1987) 'The concept of public management and the Australian state in the 1980s', *Australian Journal of Public Administration*, 46, 4: 339–53.

Yeatman, A. (1990) *Bureaucrats, Technocrats, Femocrats*, Sydney: Allen and Unwin.

Yeatman, A. (1994) *Postmodern Revisionings of the Political*, London: Routledge.

Question from Alan: I'm interested in your thoughts on how genea-logical enquiry might help us rethink the problem of welfare inequality that you refer to early in your chapter. You suggest that the documentation of this inequality should remain part of the critical reform agenda, and that governmentality is a complementary rather than an alternative form of investigation in this endeavour. However, if the basic goal of genealogy is to destabilise or undermine taken-for-granted categories of analysis, can one continue to argue for an analysis based on stable categories such as class, gender, age or ethnicity?

Response: Thanks for your question, Alan. I'm going to concentrate on what I believe to be the crux of your point: namely, 'if the basic goal of genealogy is to destabilise or undermine taken-for-granted categories of analysis, can one continue to argue for an analysis based on stable categories such as class, gender, age or ethnicity?'

I need to start by clearing the issue about genealogy. You suggest that the aim of genealogy is to 'destabilise or undermine taken-for-granted categories of analysis'. Now genealogy certainly wishes to 'render the present strange', and thus to open up spaces for imagining that things might be different. But this is not to say that destabilisation or disruption is the sole aim of genealogy. Tracing the 'conditions of possibility' which underlie current truths is, I think, a more primary task. (This is not to set genealogy apart from critique; rather to position it as a particular form of critique aspiring to a particular kind of historical understanding.)

Having said that, what of your query about whether: 'one can continue to argue for an analysis based on stable categories such as class, gender, age or ethnicity?'

In response to this, I acknowledge that poststructural thought – alongside longer-established feminist positions – has certainly asked us to consider carefully our use of global categories. However, I think it's important to disentangle what *is* from what is *not* being said here.

Starting with what *is* being asserted, two things stand out (and they are by no means unique to poststructural, let alone genealogical, analysis). First, it is argued that it is not acceptable to use categories such as class or gender as reductionist tools of explanation. That is, it is not defensible to claim that the welfare state was deliberately designed as an instrument of class oppression and/or that the great majority of its operations can be traced to that fact. Equally, any claim that gender is the principle around which all other forms of oppression are organised, and in reference to which they can be explained, is ruled out of court.

Second, it is maintained that categories such as class, gender, ethnicity, etc., cannot be used as undifferentiated descriptors. That is, they cannot be used as categories which assume that all subjects included within them possess some kind of shared identity. This point has, again, long been recognised in feminist accounts which have worried about the meaning of the word 'woman' and emphasised how gender is mediated by class, ethnicity, age, health and a host of other variables.

What then is *not* being said? Or put another way, on what occasions might a poststructuralist either continue to use these categories or (as I actually argued) recognise the force and usefulness of other traditions which choose to do so? In thinking about the answer to your question, I have come up with three such instances.

First, it is clear that poststructuralists, *qua* poststructuralists, are very concerned with the ways in which general categories are created through discursive practices. So to the extent that official and popular discourses deploy categories based on binary oppositions such as male and female, black and white, working and middle class, poststructural analysis must deal with these categories and their effects. (To recognise that such oppositions are 'imaginary' is, of course, not to take them lightly or to ignore their real material effects.)

Second, poststructuralists may agree with writers in mainstream policy traditions that categories such as class and gender are useful referents as far as the distributional impacts of policy are concerned. It seems, for example, perfectly appropriate to point out that the introduction of a goods and services tax (GST) will benefit capital against labour and 'professional' against 'working' classes. And when we consider the debate on changes to the laws governing abortion, it is clear that these changes affect women more than men. The point is not that these categories 'explain everything': a GST will differentially affect self-employed, contract and tenured labour; abortion law reform impacts differently on Catholic and pro-choice women, and so forth. The point rather, is that certain broad traditional distinctions may provide the best point of departure in these instances.

Finally, there may well be times when global categories remain indispensable to the explanation of events. I am thinking, for example, of the recent struggle over waterside reform in Australia and the coal miners' strike in the UK. It is hard to imagine any kind of analysis that does not take account of the clash between the interests of capital and labour. To be sure, the interests involved were not stable. Participants in the struggle were not necessarily united or representative of class interests. People took sides and this was not necessarily along class lines. All this poststructuralist (and other) accounts would want to point out. But my point is that without the global categories in the first place this kind of discussion could not proceed.

I hope I have gone at least part of the way to answering your question. In brief: poststructural accounts refuse to use global categories as reductionist tools of explanation and/or undifferentiated descriptors. But they treat the social binaries attached to global categories seriously, may choose to point to the impacts of certain policies along global lines, and may even acknowledge the salience of global categories as analytical starting points in certain instances.

Question from Ian: When you use the phrase 'a significant shift in the nature of the participatory bonds which constitute and join people as common members of a shared socio-political order' is this referring to another 'political rationality of rule' or a language/practice which expresses the ethos of self-governing community, etc.? What lies behind this question is the more philosophical question about whether the poststructural focus on 'governmentality' entails an epistemological displacement of the 'normative'.

Response: Before answering the 'question behind your question', I will respond to your initial query. You ask whether I am conceptualising a different 'political rationality of rule' or a 'language/practice which expresses the ethos of self-governing community' when I refer to the shift from welfarism to advanced liberalism.

The answer is both of these. Rose and Miller (1992) describe political rationalities as the 'changing discursive fields' in which the exercise of political power is justified. They go on to say that political rationalities embody a moral dimension which is concerned with the terms and conditions under which power may be rightfully exercised; an epistemological component which sets out particular understandings of governance and explains why certain things should (or should not) be subject to formal governance, and a distinctive idiom through which these understandings and justifications are discussed and circulated (ibid.: 175). Drawing from this we can say that the 'languages and practices which express the ethos of the self-governing community' are part of a political rationality (advanced liberalism) in which an understanding of individuals, communities and the economy as 'naturally' self-regulating entities justifies state intervention only in so far as it promotes those self-regulatory characteristics.

To turn to your question about whether the poststructural focus on 'governmentality' entails an epistemological displacement of the 'normative'. This needs to be answered in two ways: first, in relation to the preferences and practices of governmentality theorists; second, in relation to the notion of governance.

Governmentality theorists aim to explicate rather than evaluate governing rationalities. While they may agree that certain forms of governance are more or less coercive or more or less fair, such issues are not their prime concern. Despite this, governmentality theorists have a recognisable normative position. Most obviously, they are attached to critique as a 'troubling of truth' (O'Malley et al. 1997: 507). Questioning orthodoxy is valued because it opens spaces whereby we can consider 'the limits we may go beyond' (Foucault 1992: 309). Related to this, governmentality theorists have been particularly concerned to 'trouble truth' in areas where expert knowledges define and produce people in ways which are, in some sense, restrictive or harmful: in the orthodoxies of madness, criminality, sexuality, medicine and poverty, for example.

Turning, then, to the notion of governance. Is there something about this notion which necessarily displaces normative questions? At one level, this appears to be so. Within the governmentality frame, ideals such as social justice or democracy are discursive constructs which serve particular governmental ends. In this respect, governmentality theory treats all values as equal. Put another way, it is the relationship to governance rather than the merits of different value positions which is the issue. To this extent normative questions are irrelevant. Notions relating to the 'participatory citizen', for example, would, in this respect, score no guernsey over those relating to the 'self-regarding citizen'.

At another level, governmentality theory does not displace normative questions and may even, in certain instances, enhance their importance. Two arguments are relevant here. First, there is nothing about the governmentality frame which denies that different systems of governance have 'better' or 'worse' results according to some measure of the good society. Second, the governmentality approach does not suggest that ethical codes and preferences are reducible to, or an artefact of, governance – simply that they are deployed (and shaped) by governance. With this in mind we can suggest that ethical/normative issues have, as it were, a semi-autonomous state as far as any particular set of governmental practices is concerned, and can – for better or worse – be brought to bear on those practices. Their importance is thereby evident.

Systematic thinking about normative preferences traditionally belongs to social and political philosophy where antifoundationalism questions any supposition that normative differences can be resolved by an appeal to the universal good. Here, as in poststructuralism, contemporary developments reframe but do not displace normative questions.

References

Foucault, M. (1992) in M. Poster, *Michel Foucault, Philosopher*, New York: Routledge.
O'Malley, P., Weir, R. and Shearing, C. (1997) 'Governmentality, criticism and politics', *Economy and Society,* 26, 4: 501–17.
Rose, N. and Miller, P. (1992) 'Political power beyond the state: problematics of government', *British Journal of Sociology*, 43, 2: 173–205.

Question from Janice: You identify an enduring nexus between work and welfare in public welfare social policies. I'd be interested in your elaborating on the role of work in operating as a criterion for inclusion into or exclusion from the moral community of full and equal citizens. Is there a nexus between prudential activity, with regard to work, and citizenship, particularly in terms of the requirement of the responsible citizen that they be active in preparing themselves – for example, via the acquisition of skills and/or credentials – to be able and available to participate in the economy? Is this a reconfiguration of the nineteenth century notion of the deserving and undeserving poor – the responsible citizen who has taken action to develop marketable skills being 'deserving', in contrast to the irresponsible individual who has not been similarly proactive and is therefore undeserving of the social/community support extended to citizens?

Response: Janice, your line of thought has triggered one of my own. I will deal with mine first (apologies!) and then return to your enquiry. My preamble relates to the work–welfare nexus and changing conceptions of work.

The work-welfare nexus I talked about in the chapter existed from at least the nineteenth century on. It related, rather practically and mundanely, to the state's desire to restrict support to those 'genuinely' in need: that is, to those whose causes of need were endorsed by officials. Married women or children were included in this calculation as dependants. While the reasons for being 'genuinely' without work included sickness and old age, beliefs concerning the idleness of the labouring classes produced the principle of less eligibility.

Paradoxically, one of the reasons that less eligibility was so important as a policy instrument in the nineteenth century was that the work performed by the labouring classes was recognised to be arduous, tough and unsafe. As industrialisation took hold, the harshness of factory discipline and the danger of working in the mines was widely depicted in contemporary writings, where descriptions of work reproduced and reflected prevailing distinctions between the 'rough' and the 'gentle' classes. Industrial labour was cast in instrumental terms: it had to be done to earn subsistence. By the same token, it was something to be avoided if possible – hence the emphasis on class discipline and less eligibility.

In contrast, late twentieth-century westerners have become familiar with the discourse of 'work as self-fulfilment' and/or 'moral citizenship'. Here the insecure and arduous nature of many low-paid jobs is ignored in favour of general exhortations about active participation. This increases the unequal position of subjects through the deployment of a general or inclusive language in the face of structural difference. The effects of this are rendered the more perverse by the continued operation of less eligibility. In its current form, it produces a number of measures which ensure that people who might reasonably desist from work (because it is low paid, hazardous, insecure, detrimental to health, etc.) are either forced to do so or penalised financially if they do not.

To return to your question. You ask whether there is 'a nexus between prudential activity with regard to work and citizenship' in so far as citizens are enjoined to be 'active in preparing themselves for participation in the economy'. This trend is, indeed, part of the current repositioning of work mentioned above. In your chapter you describe the forward-looking preparation, the constant preparedness to obtain new skills or credentials, which this involves. To behave in this way is, as you suggest, to be 'responsible'. This particular rendering of responsibility is linked to an obligation both to the community (being productive, not being a burden on the state and so on) and to the self (achieving full potential, etc.). To repeat: both are underpinned by expectations relating to participation in paid work (and/or preparation to that end).

This way of thinking about responsibility, citizenship and productivity has meant that deserving/undeserving judgements have given way to a 'competitive/non-competitive' mode of assessment. This denotes more than a shuffling of deckchairs. Both the criteria and the rationale relating to the respective judgements are different. The deserving/undeserving distinction separated the worthy from the unworthy on the basis of their moral behaviour, cleanliness and industry. The distinction was made to determine who had a rightful claim for charitable or state support. In contrast, the competitive/non-competitive distinction separates the worthy from the unworthy on the basis of their skills, attitudes and current employment status. This time the distinction is made in relation to participation in the productive life of the community.

The competitive/non-competitive distinction is more inclusive and trickier than its older counterpart: more inclusive as it applies across the community rather than to the indigent class; trickier because the 'capacity to compete' provides both the grounds and the rationale for the distinction. With competition recast as an end in itself, the circle is complete.

Chapter 3

Higher education policy and the learning citizen

Janice Dudley

It is no mere coincidence that the titles of both the UK's Dearing Report (*Higher Education in the Learning Society*) and Australia's West Review (*Learning for Life*) are based on the notion of life-long learning. This organising principle – variously, 'lifelong learning', 'learning for life' and 'the learning society – is a recasting of the privileging of the economic that has been characteristic of OECD countries since the late 1970s.

Since at least the early 1980s, public policy in Australia and the UK has been dominated by the discourses of neo-liberalism and neo-classical economics. Referred to in the UK as 'Thatcherism' and in Australia as 'economic rationalism' (Pusey 1991), in the 1990s it has been reconfigured as 'globalisation' – a grand narrative of incorporation into a global capitalist economy. Globalisation is a form of economic fundamentalism, an absolutist closed discourse which privileges 'the market' – an international capitalist market place of free trade, unfettered by national regulation. It is this 'neutral' global market which becomes the paramount organising principle to which all societies must thus become subject.

In response, the welfare state becomes the competition state (Cerny 1990: 205), the discursive imperatives of globalisation requiring that the state direct its priorities towards international economic competitiveness. Yeatman (1990: 102) describes the coherent set of policy prescriptions and programmes generated by the competition state as 'metapolicy', whilst Marginson (1993: xii) uses the term 'metanarrative'.

Education policy in particular, has been directed towards constructing citizens whose subjectivities – that is, their sense of identity, their understandings of and orientations to the world – are in accord with these imperatives, and who will therefore contribute to enhancing the competitiveness of the nation's economy in the international capitalist market place.

Modern citizenship is constituted by the terms upon which the subject is normatively incorporated into the imagined political and social community. The conditions or character of that citizenship, therefore, is fundamental to the nature of the relationship between the citizens and the state. In this chapter, I am concerned with the ways in which higher education policy in both Australia and the UK have attempted to effect a particular construction of the citizen – as an economic subject articulated into an internationally competitive Australian or British economy. Education is an institution concerned with constituting and constructing particular forms of political and social subjects, and particularly since the advent of mass education, particular constructions of political and social citizens. The focus of this chapter is not the overt concern of education for citizenship – civics and the citizenship education which has been the focus of resurgent interest in both Australia and the UK in recent years (*Education for Active Citizenship*, 1988; *Active Citizenship Revisited*, 1991; *Whereas the People: Civics and Citizenship Education*, 1994; *The Discovering Democracy School Materials Project*, 1997; *Encouraging Citizenship*, 1990). Rather, my discussion will concern itself with the discursive construction, through education, of subjects who can best contribute to the order, security and prosperity of the state. I shall draw upon Foucault's work on both the analysis of discourse and on governmentality, or the rationalities of government.

Citizenship and the practices of advanced liberal governance

In liberal theory, the political community is an independent self-determining community of rational sovereign individuals who consent, via a 'social contract', to constitute a polity, or community of governance. As this community of governance is an independent self-determining community of citizens, the characteristics necessary for citizenship are independence, self-sufficiency, responsibility and rationality. In contrast to premodern or traditional notions in which divine or natural law constituted political legitimacy, the modern liberal polity is deemed to be both secular and rational and is based upon the sovereignty or autonomy of individual citizens. Modern liberal citizenship is similarly secular and rational and is grounded upon the citizen as the bearer of rights. The most significant of these rights is liberty. Freedom, and especially negative freedom[1] is an enduring strand in liberalism. The centrality of the freedom of the individual citizen necessitates limitations upon the state and the extent to which it controls or 'intrudes' directly into the lives of citizens. Hence rule or government through highly directive regulation or coercion is incompatible with liberal principles. As autonomy and agency are central to liberalism, therefore, government must needs be achieved through the agency, freedom and autonomy of citizens (see also Rose 1993; Barry *et al.* 1996). Hence to achieve the particular policy outcomes that are deemed essential to the good order, prosperity, stability and security of the polity – and hence of the citizens themselves – the citizen needs to develop those particular citizenship subjectivities likely to ensure behaviour in accordance with policy objectives. Barry *et al.* (1996: 7) refer to the late twentieth-century 'form of government based around the exercise of freedom' as advanced liberalism.

The subjectivities of citizenship are therefore constituted by the individual's normative incorporation into the community of liberal governance. As the community of governance is a form of the social contract, effectively constituting social solidarity, social coherence and social closure, the subjectivities of citizenship constitute the conditions of the social contract. Particular discursive understandings of civic virtue – the obligations of the citizen, whether these be political, economic, social – are normalising. In other words, citizenship requires conformity to particular norms, practices and behaviours, which are themselves determined by the terms of the dominant discourse.

In his later work Foucault was concerned with what he termed 'the conduct of conduct' (Burchell *et al.* 1991) or 'the government of the self by the self' and the manner in which both the management, or government, of the self and the government of populations are similarly discursive.

Political government can be described as the management of populations, and in particular the population of a state. Political government is effected as policies, which are in turn effected through technologies of government. These technologies of government contribute to the shaping, or constituting, of particular forms of subjectivity in individuals thereby leading to individuals who govern their ways of thinking and their conduct in ways which foster the order, security and prosperity of the state. Thus:

political rationalities are more than just ideologies; they constitute a part of the fabric of our ways of thinking about and acting upon one another and ourselves.

(Barry *et al*. 1996: 7)

Such rationalities of government are both individualising, in that they are concerned with the subjectivity of the individual, and totalising in rendering the population both subject to and committed to the 'common good'; in other words, committed to the order, prosperity and security of the state. Under conditions of advanced liberalism, the technologies or rationalities of government have become principally the discipline of the market, a framework of competitive social relations and practices of accountability and audit.

It is important to understand that the citizen's freedom to choose, the citizen's freedom to act are central to advanced liberal forms of government – in other words, the governmentality perspective presupposes agency.

When we are governed, when our behaviour is managed, directed or conducted by others, we do not become the passive objects of a physical determination. To govern individuals is to get them to act and to align their particular wills with ends imposed on them through constraining and facilitating models of possible action. Government presupposes and requires the activity and freedom of the governed (Burchell 1991: 119).

Rather, power is exercised as a form of indirect control, through a seemingly contradictory combination of deregulation and direction: what Rose (1993: 295) refers to as 'distantiated relations of control'. Thus power is exercised according to Foucault's understanding of power as 'the *structuring* of the possible field of action by others' (Peters 1996: 82; emphasis added). Burchell (1993: 275; 1996: 28) refers to this independent action as 'autonomization' – the freedom to act within and 'according to a kind of economic enterprise model of action which pursues a competitive logic'.

Ball (1994: 54, 66) refers to this advanced liberal form of governance as 'steering at a distance'. Government policy establishes a series of framing imperatives – levels of funding, guidelines, the 'discipline' of the market, financial accountability requirements and the like – which constrain, shape and direct the free and autonomous responses of those within the system towards the objectives and priorities of government policy:

'[S]teering at a distance' [constitutes] a new paradigm of public governance [and provides] an alternative to coercive/prescriptive control. Constraints are replaced by incentives. Prescription is replaced by *ex post* accountability based upon quality or outcome assessments. Coercion is replace by self-steering – the appearance of autonomy.

(Ibid.: 54)

Education has long been a principal tool for developing in the child, the potential citizen in whom the rationality of the sovereign individual is as yet undeveloped, the rationality essential to membership of the political community (see Marginson 1997). Education is therefore concerned to inculcate in the 'proto-citizen' those forms of rationality – or subjectivities – which shape the orientations of the individual to their relationship with the state and with society. These subjectivities are discursively contingent; by that I mean that the 'character' of the good citizen, his or her orientations and the subjectivities thus privileged are those of the dominant discourse. Education is concerned to inculcate a wide range of subjectivities across all social domains; including, but not exclusively, the political, the social and the economic, but principally those forms of subjectivity that will enable the individual self to govern itself in terms of what makes a good citizen. This is of course discursively constituted. Thus education contributes to the governing of a population according to the precepts of the dominant discourse. So if the order, security and prosperity of the state are constructed as an internationally competitive economy, the good and responsible citizen ought to act in ways which foster the international competitiveness of the nation's economy.

With the developing complexity of society and the economy, higher education has been increasingly incorporated into paradigms of education for national prosperity. The particular manner in which higher education contributes to national prosperity has, with the transformation of elite forms of post secondary education into mass higher education, been reconfigured according to the neoclassical economic precepts of economic rationalism. Thus, whereas the 'traditional' role of university education (including its immediate post Second World War incarnations in both Australia and the UK) was the training of political and economic elites, at the end of the twentieth century its 'mission' is the production of well-trained and skilled intellectual workers who are able to enhance Australia's economic competitiveness in the 'knowledge economy' (see, for example, West 1998: 16).

Higher education policy in Australia, 1987–98

The restructuring of the Australian economy away from its traditional reliance upon natural resources and primary production towards one based more upon skills, particularly intellectual skills, has been the organising imperative of Australian public policy – including education policy – since the mid-1970s. The 'lucky country' was to be transformed into the 'clever country'. As I have described in more detail elsewhere (Dudley 1998), this transformation was to be achieved via the Accord, an agreement between the Labor Party in government and the Australian trade union movement (the Australian Council of Trade Unions or ACTU). The Accord was effectively a neo-corporatist model of labour and government policy cooperation with economic restructuring as its principal objective – the social wage elements of the Accord were soon marginalised. Economic restructuring was a self-evident imperative to ensure Australia's economic competitiveness in the global capitalist economy. Through the transformation of the totality of Australian society into a competition state (Cerny 1990: 205), the prosperity and security of the nation would therefore inevitably be assured.

Whilst economic restructuring via macroeconomic reform – the deregulation of the financial system and the floating of the Australian dollar – had been the policy framework of the Labor government during its first terms of office, it was after the re-election of the Hawke Labor government in 1987 that the focus of policy shifted to microeconomic reform.

Together, the Labor government and the union movement advocated a post-Fordist route to economic competitiveness in concert with a social democratic settlement between capital and labour comparable to Scandinavia and Germany. Their priorities were industry restructuring, an active rather than a reactive trade and industry policy on the part of government, investment in industry and product innovation, together with emphases on formal training and union modernisation. These post-Fordist principles are recognisable elements in the microeconomic reform policies of Labor after 1987.

The substantive concerns of the productivity, efficiency, account-ability and performance of higher education in 'respond[ing] flexibly to the requirements of economic growth' had been the terms of reference of the Commonwealth Tertiary Education Commission's *Review of Efficiency and Effectiveness in higher education* (CTEC 1986). However, as became clear when the microeconomic restruc-turing of education began, the existing policy frameworks and institutional relationships of the higher education 'industry' were perceived as impediments to maximising the potential of higher education in contributing to the task of economic restructuring.

The Dawkins reforms

In 1987 Australian higher education was a binary system of 19 universities and 46 colleges of advanced education (CAEs) together with a small number of small specialist institutions. Universities were comprehensive research and teaching institutions, and were funded accordingly, whilst CAEs had been conceived of principally as teaching institutions with a more vocational focus. However, in the 20 or so years of their existence, CAEs had extended their range of teaching activities beyond the narrowly vocational, whilst CAE academics were engaging in a wide range of research activ-ities. Although the government of the day established the broad framework of policy, through the issuing of guidelines, higher education policy and planning was conducted at arm's length from the government of the day by an expert education commission, the Commonwealth Tertiary Education Commission.

Australian higher education was certainly in need of reform. Existing policies were no longer appropriate to its changing char-acter and the needs of students. The binary divide was increasingly irrelevant (particularly the funding differential between univer-sities and CAEs), demand from 'qualified' students was burgeoning, whilst equity issues (access to and participation in higher education by so-called disadvantaged groups) seemed intractable, given the funding they received. There were repeated calls for a Committee of Inquiry comparable to the Murray Inquiry (1957) and the Martin Inquiry (1965), that would reshape higher education policy and provide a framework more relevant and appropriate to the 1990s (Anwyl 1987a, 1987b, 1987c).

After the re-election of the Hawke Labor government in 1987, there was a major and decisive restructuring of the administration of government. The most obvious expression of this was the reorganisation and amalgamation of existing government. However, more important were the changes in administrative practice: programme budgeting, a focus upon outputs rather than inputs, performance indicators, competition between sectors and programmes (Hawke 1987; Considine 1988). The efficiency of government was to be enhanced in the interests of smaller government and the economy. The changes in the structure of the Commonwealth bureaucracy were modelled upon corporate management. The dominance of this model in the 1987 reforms was reflected in Hawke's (1987: 12) media statement: 'The new structure will . . . provide the opportunity for improved corporate management processes . . .'.

The discourse of these reforms of the 'machinery of government' was not *public service* but *management* of the business of government (see also Emy and Hughes 1991: 401–33). Their objectives were efficiency and an enhanced capacity to implement the government's policies of economic restructuring, and greater competitiveness in the international capitalist market place, through the Commonwealth bureaucracy's 'responsiveness' to its ministers.

This reorganisation of the Commonwealth bureaucracy marked the second phase of a fundamental reorientation of the administration of government which the Hawke government had been progressively implementing since its election in 1983 (Marshall 1988: 22). The goals of the policy had been articulated in the 1983 White Paper, *Reforming the Australian Public Service*. These goals were the greater responsiveness of the public service to the policy goals of government and a renewed emphasis on the primacy of ministers with respect to both policy and policy implementation:

> The objectives of the Government's proposals are to develop an administration that:
> * is more responsive and accountable to Ministers and the Parliament
> * is more efficient and effective . . . [with] a much closer involvement of Ministers in decisions.
>
> (Dawkins 1983: 1, 2)

Although the restructuring was argued to be based upon the Westminister principles of democratic and accountable government, the government's desire for greater control could be interpreted in terms of its need for more rapid and effective implementation of its policy objectives.

The new Minister for Employment, Education and Training[2] (John Dawkins) initiated fundamental change to the organisation goals and management of higher education. The binary divide was abolished and a Unified National System (UNS) established. The rationale for the reforms were:

> Consistent with the Government's objective of excellence in higher education, measures will be implemented to encourage institutions to be efficient, flexible and responsive to changing national needs. These will include:
> * measures to make more productive use of institutional resources and facilities, including institutional consolidations and more systematic credit transfer arrangements;
> * greater targeting of resources at the institutional level and improved institutional management;
> * increased flexibility and incentives for performance for both institutions and individual staff; and
> * encouragement of an environment of productive competition between higher education institutions.
>
> (Dawkins 1988: 10–11)

A number of themes was clearly evident in the proposed reforms. First, education was reconceptualised principally in terms of its contribution to economic restructuring and national economic competitiveness – education's role in the economy was the 'production' of skilled workers who were to contribute to the successful repositioning of the Australian economy in global capitalism as 'the clever country' (ibid.: 8, 17–18, 31–2). Thus emphasis on future planning and growth in the system was to focus upon developing the 'defined priority areas' of engineering, information technology, business administration, economics, management, Asian studies and technology-based courses: the 'likely future needs of the economy and the labour market' (ibid.: 17).

Second, the expansion of participation and the focus upon greater equity in the system and access of previously underrepresented groups (so called 'disadvantaged groups') to higher education was presented as an issue of human capital: barriers to participation needed to be removed in order that the full productive potential of the nation's population could be directed towards the country's economic priorities (ibid.: 12, 17, 20–1, 53–60). This perspective had been explicitly articulated in the earlier *Skills for Australia*:

> A society which does not respond to the needs of its disad-vantaged groups will incur the heavy socio-economic costs of under-developed and under-utilised human resources.
>
> . . .
>
> This is not simply a matter of meeting social objectives related to equity. Rather it is *an economic argument about increasing the pool of human resources available.* . . .
>
> (Dawkins and Holding, 1987: 15–16, emphasis added)

However, this increased participation was to be achieved without additional funding from government. Rather, it was to be achieved through a combination of efficiency gains in the higher education sector ('industry') itself, and higher levels of 'contribution' from the beneficiaries and clients of education – that is, graduates and industry (Dawkins 1988: 10–12, 27, 29–32). With education recon-stituted as a private rather than a public or collective good, the reintroduction of tuition fees (which had been abolished by the Whitlam Labor government in 1974) effected the 'user pays' principle (Wran 1988). The Higher Education Contribution Scheme (HECS) was a system of tuition fees of approximately 20 per cent of real costs, with the options of 'up-front' payment or deferred payment through the taxation system. These forms of 'privatisation' together with the increasing numbers of fee-paying overseas students (the developing industry of the export of education services) were to shift the burden – not only of growth but also of public higher education as a whole – from government or the state to individuals and the private sector. Efficiency and an entrepre-neurial culture were to be enhanced via the introduction of competi-tion for research funding and also for teaching resources, the latter funded by a small but significant reduction in operating grants.

A fourth element was the devolution to individual institutions of greater control over, and responsibility for, their spending and admin-istration, and also for achieving the 'agreed priorities' which were to be negotiated between government and individual institutions via 'Institutional Profiles' (Dawkins 1988: 71–8). In addition, institutions were exhorted to introduce 'streamlined' and efficient models of corporate management and 'flexible' staffing (ibid.: 101–13).

The emphasis upon quality

With the establishment of the Unified National System, Australian higher education moved from an elite to a mass system. The outcomes orientation of the new arrangements and the accountability requirements embedded in the new institutional relationships between government and universities, OECD concerns for quality and the international quality movement – for example, the International Network of Quality Assurance in Higher Education (Vidovich and Porter 1997: 235) – were factors which contributed to and influenced the focus upon 'quality' in Australian higher education in the 1990s. In 1991, a process for establishing a system of quality audits was initiated by the Minister for Employment, Education and Training. The Higher Education Council (HEC), the departmental higher education advisory body, produced a series of discussion papers to enable 'stakeholders', including students, academic staff, university administrations and the Australian Vice-Chancellors' Committee (AVCC), to participate in shaping the terms and processes of the reviewing of the quality of Australian higher education.

The process was to consist of the competitive allocation of 'quality funds' (additional to institutions' operating grants) on the basis of the effectiveness of their quality assurance mechanisms:

> Universities would be invited (not compelled) to participate ... the key features being an institutional portfolio of self-assessment, visits by a review committee and the use of nationally available data. In addition to placing universities in performance bands (not individual rankings) which would determine rewards, the Committee [for Quality Assurance in Higher Education] would provide advice to universities, disseminate best practices and monitor the benefits of allocated funds after three years.
>
> (Vidovich and Porter 1997: 237)

The three-year cycle of quality audits (1993–5) contributed to the growing competitive orientation of the UNS, both within institutions and between individual institutions. The rankings, which on each occasion favoured the older, larger and longer-established research universities in each State, appeared to provide legitimating support for arguments in favour of concentrating the limited research funding available in 'premier' or elite institutions.

Coalition policies

In 1996, the Australian Labor Party (ALP), which had governed Australia since 1983 under Prime Minister Hawke and Prime Minister Keating, was defeated and a Liberal/National Party coalition[3] government was elected under the leadership of John Howard. Coalition policies were to eliminate the 'bureaucratic regulation', 'intrusion', 'government red-tape' and corporate managerialism of the Labor years, and enhance the autonomy, flexibility and choice of institutions, together with support for greater 'diversity' in the system. Substantive changes, however, were more of degree than of kind. Universities were required both to become more efficient and to ensure higher levels of funding from private sources as operating grants were to decline by 4 per cent over the four-year period 1996–2000, whilst, continuing the policies of its Labor predecessor, the government declined to index university operating grants in order to provide funding for staff salary increases, thereby ensuring effective additional declines in operating funding.

The reconstitution of education as a private rather than a collective responsibility was furthered through changes to HECS and student support programmes. From 1997, programmes of study were differentiated into three bands with differing levels of HECS liability, based on the cost of provision and perceptions of the greater private benefit students would receive in their later working lives[4] whilst the repayment threshold was reduced to below average weekly earnings. Levels of student support declined in real terms to below the statistical poverty line and the age of independence was raised from 22 to 25 years. In addition, with the removal of the legislative impediment to enrolling fee-paying Australian undergraduates,[5] universities were to be free from 1998 to enrol private Australian students. In spite of the growth in real terms of non-government sources of funding, the effect of the decline in government funding was no net gain for institutions; rather, the increasing proportion of university budgets acquired from non-government sources meant a progressive shift from public provision of education to private purchase.

Learning for Life: review of higher education financing and policy

Learning for Life – the West Review – was appointed in January 1997 by the then Minister, Senator Amanda Vanstone, to develop a policy and funding framework for higher education in the twenty-first century. It was required to

> undertake a broad ranging review of the state of Australia's higher education sector, the effectiveness of the sector in meeting Australia's social, economic, cultural and scientific needs, and the developments which are likely to shape the provision of higher education in the next two decades.

Whilst there was no 'wish to limit the scope of the Review committee's work', the Committee was to make its recommendations in the context of:

> the level and nature of industry demand for higher education graduates and higher education research, and the contribution that graduates and research conducted within higher education institutions make to the competitiveness of Australian industry;
>
> . . .
>
> policy and practice in public sector financing and management, including the increased emphasis on competition, contestability and competitive neutrality principles;

and finally:

> [i]n developing its recommendations, the government expects that the Review Committee will pay particular attention to the need to ensure that:
> *   public funds for higher education teaching and research are used efficiently and effectively, and appropriate accountability mechanisms are in place . . .
>
> (West 1998: 177–9)

Framing its recommendations in a commitment to lifelong learning and a revisioning of Australian society as a 'learning society', the Review recommended a shift from the existing regulated quasi-market relationships between universities and between universities and the state to a more fully competitive and market-based approach – 'a policy framework that is driven by the needs and preferences of those who use the services of universities' (ibid.: 15).

This was to be effected, first, by a shift to student-centred funding, through funding following students' choices of programmes, courses and institutions; second, by ensuring the 'responsiveness of higher education research to the needs of the users of that research' (ibid.); and third, by establishing the conditions for the development of Australian higher education as a 'world class . . . industry' (ibid.).

The principal and most contested recommendation was that school leavers and mature age students who had not previously undertaken post secondary study would qualify for a 'lifelong learning entitlement' (ibid.: 24). These 'consumers' (students) would 'purchase' education services from a provider (existing public universities, existing private higher education institutions or new private institutions, whether Australian or international) using their financial resources (their learning entitlements). In other words, the model of funding proposed was that of a voucher system. Cash or real money could be used as an alternative to a voucher if the student had 'expended' their entitlement (for example, if an individual wished to undertake a second undergraduate degree).

At the same time, a framework of financial accountability to students – consumer protection and complaints procedures comparable to existing models of consumer protection in the retail economy – would be established, together with the provision of data enabling consumers to compare institutions. Such measures would ensure the efficient operation of the market through consumers being fully informed and so able to differentiate between the 'products' being offered by particular educational service providers. Finally, some form of safety net would ensure the continuing existence of those 'disciplines deemed to be in the national interest, and for which all provide-based options for preserving those disciplines have been exhausted' (ibid.: 28).

The Review was concerned to establish policy principles which would eliminate from the higher education industry 'the perverse incentive structures, inflexibility, restrictions on competition and entry to the market' (ibid.: 21). Thus its recommendations were based on the need for universities to develop a 'direct financial relationship' (ibid.: 24) with students in order to ensure that the disciplines of such market relationships would ensure the competitive behaviour of institutions.

University research practices were similarly argued to be in need of the stimulus of competition, in order to enhance their capacity to service the necessary developments in Australia of the high-technology industries and associated skilled workforce essential to 'an outwardly oriented, knowledge based economy' (ibid.: 16). A student-centred focus was again recommended: institutions were to compete nationally for research students. Student mobility and choice would enhance efficiency and make the most and best use of limited research resources.

Finally, establishing a world-class higher education industry in Australia would be achieved through competition between existing institutions and between public and private providers. The Review was highly critical of existing regulatory arrangements, arguing, first, that they were limiting the capacity of institutions to respond flexibly and innovatively to their consumers and to changing education market circumstances and opportunities; second, that they inhibited the development of improved management practices in universities; and finally, that together with 'subsidies' for 'public' universities, they were effectively preventing the establishment of private institutions and so breaching principles of competitive neutrality.

The Review was blunt in its message to institutions regarding its vision of the Australian university of the twenty-first century:

> Sooner rather than later, universities will need to address the essential incompatibility of a view of the world based on collegial decision making and an alternative view based on executive decision making and reflected in the size and style of operation of most business boards.
>
> Ultimately, the internal decision making processes of universities will be reformed only by universities themselves. We note that the imperative for universities to review and modify their decision making structures will intensify as their environment changes. Failure to address the inflexibilities of their current decision making processes will mean that institutions will not be well placed to operate under any financing and regulatory framework which increases competition among institutions and gives greater influence to student choice.
>
> (Ibid.: 23, 24)

The West Review presented its final report to the then Minister, Dr David Kemp, in April 1998. However, between April and the announcement in September of an October election, the Minister was preoccupied with the troublesome semi-privatisation of the

Commonwealth Employment Service (CES) into the Jobs Network: a network of private and community employment service providers operating on commercial user-pays principles, together with a significantly 'downsized' and non-comprehensive government service (Employment Australia). Hence, other than rejection of the voucher proposals and a broad endorsement of the emphasis upon institutional flexibility and 'responsiveness' to student and industry needs, there was no comprehensive response by the government to the recommendations of *Learning for Life.*

In spite of the attempts of a coalition of the Australian Vice-Chancellors' Committee (AVCC), higher education unions and students to establish higher education funding as an election issue, the 1998 election was fought on the issue of the introduction of a Goods and Services Tax: the government claimed that the higher education sector would receive substantial financial benefit from the introduction of the new tax regime, but there were no funding initiatives or shifts in policy focus.

After the re-election of the Liberal/National Party coalition to government and the reappointment of Dr David Kemp to the newly streamlined Ministry of Education, Training and Youth Affairs, the Minister indicated that he would be embarking on discussions with the university sector regarding responses to the West proposals. Priorities were reportedly the two issues of the relationship between funding and student choice, and lifelong learning (Osmond 1998; Healy and Richardson 1998).

Whilst the government in its first term of office may have rejected the West Review's voucher proposals, there has been a continuing shift in focus to outcomes measures and performance indicators, including student satisfaction (for example, the Course Experience Questionnaire or CEQ), graduation rates, graduate employment (for example, the Graduate Destinations Survey) (Illing 1998; Moodie 1998; Spencer 1998). Such information is likely to establish the framework of publicly available institutional data recommended by *Learning for Life* as necessary for the lifelong learning entitlement model envisaged in the Review.

'Steering at a distance'

For all their faults, the model of policy making in education in both Britain and Australia had, since the Second World War, been consultative, pluralist committees of inquiry. However, in Australia, after the public service reforms of the mid-1980s, the policy focus shifted to the Minister and his or her department. Lingard *et al.* (1993) refer to this as the 'ministerialisation' of education policy, and certainly the reforms of the higher education sector demonstrated the potential for speed and responsiveness of policy implementation when policy was sourced from the Minister's office. The argument for policy processes of 'ministerialisation' is a good deal more convincing because the minister at the time – John Dawkins, Minister for Employment, Education and Training – was a particularly energetic and directive protagonist of his government's reform proposals, not only in higher education but also in schooling and vocational education.

However, the character of the reform proposals themselves, and the nature of the relationship envisaged between institutions and government, would on a first reading appear to provide a high level of autonomy and independence for those within the system, be they institutions, institutional actors, individual academics or individual students:

> The Government will also ensure that institutions are free to manage their own resources without unnecessary intervention, while at the same time remaining clearly accountable for their decisions and actions. . . . Institutions will be free to establish their own priorities and develop their strengths, to accredit their own courses, to develop a broader base of funding support and to introduce more flexible staffing arrangements. Unnecessary restrictions will be lifted . . .
>
> The higher education system currently costs the Australian taxpayer around $2800m each year. Accountability for the expenditure of these resources will be a shared responsibility.
>
> The Commonwealth will identify national goals and priorities for the higher education system, and ensure that system-wide resources are allocated more effectively in accordance with those priorities. At a more detailed level, the Commonwealth will adopt new funding mechanisms that give maximum autonomy to institutions in the management of their resources, within a framework of agreed institutional goals and objectives. The performance of institutions against these goals will be a key factor in determining their future levels of income from Commonwealth sources.
>
> (Dawkins 1988: 10)

The autonomy and freedom of institutions were, however, constrained by the Commonwealth's 'national goals and priorities' and the terms of the accountability required of higher education by the government. Arguably, therefore, these policies constitute a case more of 'steering at a distance' (Ball 1994: 54, 66) than of autonomy and independence.

Whilst coalition policies claimed to be less intrusive and to eschew the 'corporate managerialism' of Labor's bureaucratic approach to policy and accountability (Meredyth 1998: 20–2),[6] the steering afforded by its funding policies continued the patterns of governance initiated under Labor. Of course, the commitment to self-management in accord with government priorities is on occasion in need of greater direction, as evidenced by the comments of the Minister, Dr David Kemp, in a 1998 paper in which he criticised university staff recruitment and promotion practices, university library purchasing practices and the size and character of university governing bodies.

Thus, whereas the specifics of policy may have varied between Labor and Liberal governments, the substantive policy objectives have remained the same: that is, enhancing Australia's competitiveness in the international economy – whilst the governmental practices of advanced liberalism are also essentially similar. Labor and Liberal/Coalition policies differ principally in the extent and emphases on the discursive constraints or, in other words, in the extent and emphases on the particular rationalities of market relations, accountability and audit. Thus, whereas Labor policies would appear to accord more closely to the post-Fordist 'Left Moderniser' model of Brown and Lauder (1996), the Liberal/Coalition policies would seem more closely aligned to the neo-Fordist pattern (see Table 3.1).

Britain: higher education under New Labour

The Dearing Review of higher education (*Higher Education in the Learning Society*) was established with cross-party support in May 1996 to provide a vision for British higher education in the twenty-first century. It presented its report in July 1997 soon after the election of Tony Blair's New Labour government. Its terms of reference were broad and encompassed:

Table 3.1 Post-Fordist possibilities: alternative models of national development

Fordism	Neo-Fordism	Post-Fordism
Protected national markets.	Global competition through productivity gains, cost-cutting (overheads, wages).	Global competition through innovation, quality, value-added goods and services.
	Inward investment attracted by 'market flexibility' (reduce the social cost of labour, trade union power).	Inward investment attracted by highly skilled labour force engaged in 'value added' production/services.
	Adversarial market orientation: remove impediments to market competition. Create 'enterprise culture'. Privatisation of the welfare state.	Consensus-based objectives: corporatist 'industrial policy'. Cooperation between government, employers and trade unions.
Mass production of standardised products/ low skill, high wage.	Mass production of standardised products/low skill, low wage 'flexible' production and sweatshops.	Flexible production systems/small batch/niche markets; shift to high-wage, high-skilled jobs.
Bureaucratic hierarchical organisations.	Leaner organisations with emphasis on 'numerical' flexibility.	Leaner organisations with emphasis on 'functional' flexibility.
Fragmented and standardised work tasks.	Reduce trade union job demarcation.	Flexible specialisation/ multiskilled workers.
Mass standardised (male) employment.	Fragmentation/polarisation of labour force. Professional 'core' and 'flexible' workforce (i.e. part-time, temps, contract, portfolio careers).	Maintain good conditions for all employees. Non-'core' workers receive training, fringe benefits, comparable wages, proper representation.
Divisions between managers and workers/low trust relations/collective bargaining.	Emphasis on 'managers' right to manage'. Industrial relations based on low-trust relations.	Industrial relations based on high trust, high discretion, collective participation.
Little 'on the job' training for most workers.	Training 'demand' led/little use of industrial training policies.	Training as a national investment/state acts as strategic trainer.

Source: Brown and Lauder 1996: 6

the purposes, shape, structure, size and funding of higher education, including support for students, [which] should develop to
meet the needs of the United Kingdom over the next 20 years.
(Dearing 1997: Chairman's Foreword, para. 1)

However, it was clear from the terms of reference that higher education had become subsumed into the economic – particularly in
regard to enhancing the international competitiveness of the British
economy. For example:

there should be maximum participation in initial higher education by young and mature students and in lifetime learning by
adults, having regard to the needs of individuals, the nation and
the future labour market;

. . .

learning should be increasingly responsive to employment needs
and include the development of general skills, widely valued
in employment.
(Ibid.: Terms of Reference)

Whilst acknowledging that

higher education continues to have a role in the nation's social,
moral and spiritual life; in transmitting citizenship and culture
in all its variety; and in enabling personal development for the
benefit of individuals and society as a whole,
(Ibid.: Terms of reference, Annex A)

the context of the review was principally of

increasingly competitive international markets [with] the prolif-
eration of knowledge, technological advances and the information revolution . . . [where] many of our international competitors are aiming to improve the contribution their higher
education systems make to their economic performance;

. . .

through scholarship and research, higher education [would
provide] a national resource of knowledge and expertise for the
benefit of our international competitiveness and quality of life,

and [provide] a basis for responding to social and economic change through innovation and lifelong learning.

(Ibid.)

Recommendations

The review was comprehensive and detailed, making 93 recommendations. The principle informing the conclusions of the review was the integration of Universities and higher education with and for the economy. This objective was to be achieved through widening access to and increasing participation in both higher education and further education; through a new focus and higher priority being accorded to teaching and learning in higher education; through enhanced quality assurance practices together with the production of appropriate data to enable students to assess individual institutions, and the development of 'a fair and robust complaints system' (Recommendation 25); and through enhancing the efficiency of university governing bodies – such efficiency was to be modelled upon the model of corporate boards, although there was also a recommendation for the mandatory inclusion of staff and student representatives together with a majority of lay persons (Recommendation 59).

However, the most significant recommendations of the review were in respect of the funding of higher education. In his Foreword the Chairman commented:

> We recognise the need for new sources of finance for higher education to respond to these problems and to provide for growth. We therefore recommend that students enter into an obligation to make contributions to the cost of their higher education once they are in work.
>
> (Ibid.: Chairman's Foreword, para. 8)

The model recommended by the review was that institutional funding should be determined by student demand for its courses: in other words, that funding should follow student choice (Recommendation 72). Dearing (1998: 34) later referred to this as 'empowering student choice'. In addition, students were to be expected to pay approximately 25 per cent of the average cost of tuition through an income-contingent deferred payment mechanism comparable to the Australian HECS model (Recommendation 79).

Dearing, in his 1998 Menzies Oration, discussed the review's recommendation in terms of partnership – partnerships between the individual and the state, partnerships between industry, government and society, as follows:

> A series of bilateral compacts to realise the potential that lies in higher education for all estates of the realm ... [offering] not only a new source of non-State income for the university but enrichment ... for academics and contact ... with the latest developments in industry and commerce.
>
> (Dearing 1998: 34)

The government's response

The Blair government was selective in its support for the Dearing recommendations, endorsing them only to the extent that they were compliant with and advanced its own agenda. The review was effectively subsumed into the government's wider programme of Lifelong Learning, which had been the focus (and title) of New Labour's pre-election education manifesto.

The immediate response was to increase participation through the removal of the existing cap on student numbers, particularly in further education and at sub-degree level, together with a focus on access. The Australian HECS style option of deferred student fees was rejected in favour a rationalisation of the existing mix of grants and loans towards a family income contingent loan scheme. There was to be no contribution to tuition fees from low-income families nor any increase in parental contribution from middle- and high-income families. The student's debt would be recouped through the taxation system when the graduate's income reached a threshold of £10,000 (Blunkett, House of Commons Hansard Debates, 23 July 1997, columns 949–51). Further initiatives were deferred until the completion of the Comprehensive Funding Review which would establish the priorities of the new government within its commitment to 'fiscal responsibility', expressed in its pre-election commitment to maintain the previous Tory government's spending limits.

The government's detailed response to the Dearing Review, *Higher Education for the 21st Century*, was released in February 1998 whilst further commitments to the funding of an additional 500,000 places in both HE and FE to achieve a target of 40 per cent participation by 2002 were announced in the context of the Chancellor's Comprehensive Funding Review in July 1998.

At the same time, the President of the Board of Trade announced an exemplar of the new funding paradigm of partnership between industry and the state: a contribution by the Wellcome Foundation of £400 million to university teaching and research in the sciences, which in partnership with government funding would result in a total of £1.1 billion for universities and national research and development (Brown, House of Commons Hansard Debates, 14 July 1998, column 191).

UK Lifelong Learning

The Blair government has placed education at the centre of its vision for the economic and social renewal of British society. It aspires to be an, indeed *the*, education government, as the following quotations demonstrate:

> Education, education, education . . . our manifesto commitment to the British people.
> > (Brown, House of Commons Debates, 14 July 1998, column 190)

> Education is the Government's number one priority. It is key to helping our business compete and giving opportunities to all.
> > (Blair 1997)

> Education is the best economic policy we have.
> > (Blair 1998)

> Learning is the key to economic prosperity – for each of us as individuals, as well as for the nation as a whole. It has a vital role to play in promoting social inclusion . . .
> > (Blunkett 1998a)

> This is why the government has put learning at the heart of its ambition.
> > (Blunkett 1998b)

Lifelong Learning provides the framework of virtually all British education policy under New Labour. UK Lifelong Learning, the programme of policies organised around this principle, includes the Adult and Community Learning Fund, Career Development

Loans, Small Firms Training Loans, Individual Learning Accounts (ILAs), Learning Direct, the University for Industry (UfI), together with the reports: *Learning for the Twenty-First Century: First Report of the National Advisory Group for Continuing Education and Lifelong Learning*; *The Learning Age: A Renaissance for a New Britain*; *Further Education for the New Millennium*; *Higher Education for the 21st Century*.

What is evident in this series of policies for Lifelong Learning in the learning society is the manner in which each is in some way structured around the principle of partnership, partnership between stakeholders – the individual, the state, the employer.

Lifelong Learning and the learning society

Lifelong Learning is the 'new consensus – of the OECD, of the European Union[7] (Avis *et al.* in Ainley 1998: 560). There are a number of elements to learning for life, or living in the learning society. First, in the context of globalisation, lifelong learning is essential for maintaining a skilled flexibly responsive workforce. This flexibility requires the constant upgrading of skills and/or the reskilling of workers in response to the rapidly and inevitably changing demands of the world economy so that, whilst workers need always to be learning, more importantly they need to develop an orientation towards learning, multiskilling, reskilling and changing employment during their working lives:

> In a 'learning society' individuals continually invest in their own human capital . . . knowledge and skills 'transferable' from one challenging project to the next in varied and flexible careers.
> The predisposition towards 'learning to learn' thus becomes the only constant in a constantly changing world.
>
> (Ainley 1998: 559, 560)

This perspective is clearly articulated in the foreword to the European Union Lifelong Learning Conference held in Manchester in May 1998 during Britain's Presidency of the European Union:

> Economic competitiveness, employment and the personal fulfil-ment of the citizens of Europe is no longer mainly based on the production of physical goods, nor will it be in the future. Real wealth creation will henceforth be linked to the production

and dissemination of knowledge and will depend first and foremost on our efforts in the field of research, education and training and on our capacity to promote innovation. This is why we must fashion a true 'Europe of Knowledge'.

This process is directly linked to the aim of developing lifelong learning which the Union has set itself . . . expressing the determination of the Union to promote the highest level of knowledge for its people through access to education and its permanent updating.

(http://www.lifelonglearning.co.uk/conference/guide01.htm)

Second, the learning society is a stakeholder society, where learning – and especially the financing of that education – is facilitated through partnerships between stakeholders. These stakeholders include, but are not limited to, the individual citizen, the citizen's family, the state, the union movement and industry. The model is one of

[s]haring responsibility with employers, employees and the community by . . . promoting new partnerships between firms, employees and trade unions.

(The Learning Age: A Summary, 1998)

The vouchers – or lifelong learning entitlements – recommended by the West and Dearing Reviews are a relatively simple expression of a partnership between the individual citizen and the state: the citizens' entitlement provides them with the resources to act independently as consumers within an education market place. However, the Independent Learning Accounts (ILAs) envisaged for New Labour's Learning Age are a sophisticated attempt to incorporate *all* potential stakeholders into the cause of enhancing the prosperity of the nation through learning. ILAs are literally accounts (bank accounts, SmartCard accounts) to which individuals, their families, their employers, their trade union, together with the state, can contribute. The citizen-learner can draw down upon this account throughout his or her life – going into debt if necessary – in order to finance chosen personal learning needs, aspirations, ambitions.

Finally, the language of the learning society is seductively of participation, agency, control over one's own life, independence and empowerment. According to the UK Lifelong Learning web site –

the Department for Education and Employment (DfEE) web site for the encouragement, promotion and development of lifelong learning – 'learning improves your . . . prospects, career, life' (http: //www/lifelonglearning.co.uk/). The tailoring of programmes to suit the unique and individual circumstance of the lifelong learner as promised by the Learning Age's Individual Learning Accounts (see, for example, the stories of Kate and George[8]) promises autonomy, opportunity, prosperity, success. Yet the language is also of responsibility and obligation: whilst lifelong learning may provide the citizen-learner with opportunities for personal development, opportunities which resonate positively with the languages of self-realisation and self-actualisation, learning for life also suggests an unending task, that learning has become a 'life sentence'. In addition, there are the languages of contract and prudentialism: partnerships are a form of contract and may be binding; they inevitably carry responsibilties together with opportunities, so that unemployment, exclusion and despair may be the lot of those who have not embraced, or at least accepted, the conditions of citizenship in the learning society.

The learning society requires that individuals be active in their own citizenship – agency, constructed principally as economic agency, has become an obligatory element of citizenship status. Thus the individual is incorporated into citizenship as an active learner-worker.

The learning society is also the OECD's 'active society' (Walters 1997) where each citizen is a worker, an 'active participant' in the community. According to the OECD:

> The basic thrust of the notion of the 'active society' is to foster economic opportunity and activity for everyone in order to combat poverty, dependency and social exclusion.
>
> (Walters 1997: 224)

The life of the community is effectively defined as work, or participation in the economy.

In both the active society and the learning society, therefore, life and citizenship are conflated with work and participation in the economy, particularly in ways which will enhance the competitiveness of the nation's economy in world markets. As learning is required for successful economic participation, so too it is required for successful participation in life. A nexus is constructed between citizenship and economic participation. Without learning and active participation as learner-workers, citizens risk their equal participation in the citizenship community. The obverse of the nexus between citizenship and economic participation is that those not actively employed or learning are necessarily diminished in their citizenship status and rights entitlements.

Conclusion

The state of the late twentieth century is the competition state. The competition state responds to the challenges of globalisation with policies which privilege the competitiveness of the nation's economy in the capitalist market place. The particular form taken by the discourses of neo-classical economics and neo-liberal politics in Australia during the 1980s and early 1990s has been termed 'economic rationalism'. Economic rationalism is centred upon economic growth, international competitiveness and post-Fordist responses to globalisation. Economically rational subjects are both consumers and producers. As consumers, the subject is the rational self-interested individual who maximises his (*sic*) and his nuclear family's economic well being – in other words, economic man. As a producer, the subject is positioned as a worker within the economy whose role is to maximise his contribution to the competitiveness of the Australian economy in the international capitalist market place.

OECD countries such as Australia and the UK are pursuing post-Fordist strategies of building knowledge economies. Education, therefore, has assumed a crucial role in enhancing the state's capacity for success. In Australia, education policy has privileged the competitive economic individual. Agency has been constituted and restricted to the economic, whilst difference has been constituted as interest, the discourse(s) of economic liberalism universalising citizens as individuals with interests. Difference has been subsumed within the subjectivity of the economic actor and constructed as a secondary characteristic ultimately reducible to an economic subjectivity. Issues of equity are reconstructed in terms of maximising human resources, productivity and competitiveness in the global market economy. The universality of citizenship entitlement is reconstructed in terms of 'mutual obligation'.

In Britain, Thatcherite policies have been replaced by New Labour's 'Learning for Life'. In the learning society the citizen is the learner-worker, upon whom the responsibility for economic competitiveness, and hence responsibility for the prosperity, social coherence and social solidarity of the nation, depends. The learning society is a 'stakeholder society' where partnerships between citizens and the state (principally but not exclusively financial) structure not only the provision of services such as education but also citizenship itself.

The learner-worker, who is both citizen-learner and citizen-worker, may have opportunities for self-development throughout life, yet the context of globalisation and its associated economic imperatives require that the worker is sentenced to learning for life. Citizenship is precarious and depends upon the individual fulfilling her or his obligations to the stakeholder partnership. The citizen must be active in contributing to the contracted partnership through learning and working. Individuals who do not contribute to the prosperity of the nation through fulfilling their citizenship obligations of productive activity risk their citizenship, their full and equal membership of the national community.

Thus the learning society – a sophisticated example of the rationalities of advanced liberal governance – effects government through agency, through freedom, through autonomy, through empowerment. The stakeholder society of the learning society is simultaneously the competition state, the contracting state and the active society where citizenship is constructed in terms of economic participation. However, the paradox of advanced liberal rationalities of government is that whilst the agency of the individual citizen is fundamental, yet it cannot be controlled – it can be constrained, it can be steered, yet uncertainty and contingency remain immanent in autonomy. In other words, it is the very autonomisation of advanced liberal forms of government – or in other words, the freedom to act – which opens up possibilities for citizenship other than as an agent of economic competitiveness articulated into globalised capitalism.

Whilst the languages of obligation and responsibility may constrain, so too the languages of possibility and opportunity may empower. The seductive languages of empowerment, hope and community embedded in the near-religious appeal of contributing to the national task of social and economic renewal through participating in the learning society may lead to unintended or unexpected outcomes. At the same time, whilst the economic reductionism of globalisation may be dominant, yet it is not uncontested.

Education constitutes but one dimension of the discursive struggle over citizenship. Therefore, education can be a site of possibility as much as it is a site of containment. Whilst economically reductionist policies may direct, shape and frame education practice, education practices are governed by a multiplicity of imperatives which are variously and at once both competing and complementary, explicit and implicit. Education policies and practices constitute a series of tensions and paradoxes, so that, for example, whilst education policies may privilege neo-classical economics and neo-liberal politics, parallel policies of citizenship education engage with difference and with articulating such ideals as cultural pluralism, indigenous reconciliation and inclusivity. Thus education policy and education practices discursively construct 'citizens' variously in terms of the economy, the democratic polity, gender, their relationship to the state, ethnicity and/or race, class, and in terms of their relationship to the non-human natural world.

Citizenship is inevitably a site both of containment and of possibility.

Notes

1 Negative freedom is the freedom of the individual from interference. However, as all individuals are moral and hence political equals, the freedom to get on with their own lives must be constrained to the extent that that freedom does not inhibit or limit the freedom of others.

2 The department was to be Education, Employment and Training; however, it became Employment, Education and Training – the Minister considered employment and participation in the economy to be the natural focus and priority of education (Dawkins 1987: 1) and hence of primary importance.

3 The Liberal Party of Australia, whilst founded upon Liberal principles in 1944 by Robert Menzies (later Sir Robert Menzies) parallels the British Conservative Party more closely than it does the Liberal Democrats. The National Party – originally the Country Party – has traditionally been the party supported by rural landowners. Thus the Liberal and National Parties are the parties of property – urban and rural.

4 *Band 1*: Arts, Humanities, Legal Studies, Social Studies/Behavioural Science, Visual/Performing Arts and Nursing;
Band 2: Mathematics, Computing, Other Health Sciences, Agriculture, Renewable Resources, Built Environment/Architecture, Sciences, Engineering, Processing and Administration, and Business or Economics;

Band 3: Law, Medicine, Medical Science, Dentistry, Dental Services, Veterinary Science.

Thus Law, whilst a relatively inexpensive course, is included in the highest rate band because of the higher than average incomes of legal practitioners.

5   An element of the Whitlam Labor government's abolition of tertiary tuition fees in 1974.

6   The antibureaucratic policy orientation of the Liberal/National Party Coalition government (Meredyth 1998: 22) is reflected in the approximately 15 per cent 'downsizing' of the Australian Public Service (APS) between the Coalition's election in 1996, and 1998. (The decline in the decade 1986–96 under Labor was approximately 24 per cent.) The Coalition's public service reforms envisage a model of an APS pared down to a 'core service' providing policy advice, whilst policy implementation and/or the delivery of services is contracted out to the private sector.

7   The role of supranational organisations such as the OECD, the World Bank and the European Union in disseminating and furthering the discourses of globalisation and economic liberalism cannot be underestimated; see, for example, Marginson (1997: 149–79); Currie and Newsome (1998); Lingard and Rizvi (1998).

8   The following – the stories of Kate and George – is an extract from the DfEE pamphlet advertising the opportunities that The Learning Age can provide for citizens:

What will the Learning Age look like?

With the University for Industry and individual learning accounts – working together with the wide range of existing education providers – the Learning Age could look something like this.

Kate and George see a trailer for the UfI Learning Hotline on TV. It focuses on businesses making more money and people improving their earning power through learning. They phone the 24-hour-a-day UfI Hotline. It puts them through to the national call centre which provides membership services, initial advice and 'signposting'.

Kate's story

Kate left school with five O levels. She recently returned to full-time work in a supermarket after her younger child started school. But she feels there is little chance of advancing.

When she calls 0800 100 900, the Careers Service adviser tells Kate about *What Learning?*, the 'taster' series on the new digital television Learning Channel.

The careers adviser sets up the Learning Account and Learning Smartcard and enrols Kate on an IT skills course – all in the comfort of her own home. Kate finds that she can do her course partly on her children's computer with its on-line access and partly by going to classes on Saturday afternoons. These classes are held at the local UfI centre run by the further education college in the local library. She can also drop in at the UfI centre at any time if she needs advice or just wants to talk things over with other learners.

Kate tells her manager about her plans. He agrees to contribute to her Learning Account if she includes spreadsheet training in her course. He also says that Kate can use the usual Tuesday morning staff training session to develop her IT skills. He asks the UfI centre to broker a tailored training package to help his accounts office team operate their recently upgraded IT system.

George's story

George runs a catering and banqueting firm. He depends on a range of suppliers for everything from food and napkins to catering staff and DJs. This is his main problem. Although he runs a tight ship and is an Investor in People, he has problems over quality of products and failure to meet deadlines.

His UfI adviser points him in the direction of *Chain Reaction*, a website with case studies of companies which have built quality into their supply chain by requiring high quality standards of suppliers.

George backs up his planning with a *Chain Reaction* CD-ROM produced by the National Training Organisation for his sector. He organises some joint courses on Total Quality Management and Just in Time principles with some of his regular suppliers. Within two months, George is ready to set quality standards and demand that suppliers keep to them.

Five years later . . .

Kate's supermarket has funded her to take NVQs in management and financial management. She has been promoted. She uses the 'learning room' at work to upgrade her skills and has persuaded her husband to enrol on a French course at the local college.

George had a tough time with the suppliers in the first few months. However he kept going, and found an electronic 'pen pal' in a similar business based in Aberdeen through his Internet links who gave him advice. Within two years, targets had been met, and all of his suppliers were on their way to Investor in People status. Expansion was slow and controlled but within five years profits had doubled, and he was employing 20 people.

(*The Learning Age: A Summary*)

References

Active Citizenship Revisited (1991) A Report by the Senate Standing Committee on Employment Education and Training, Canberra: Australian Government Publishing Service.

Ainley, P. (1998) 'Towards a learning or a certified society? Contradictions in the New Labour modernization of lifelong learning', *Journal of Education Policy*, 13, 4: 559–73.

Anwyl, J. (1987a) 'Looking beyond the binary era', *The Australian Higher Education Supplement*, 8 April: 14.

Anwyl, J. (1987b) 'Sliding towards anarchy in higher education planning', *FAUSA News*, 6 May: 8, 9.

Anwyl, J. (1987c) *Adjusting to the Post Binary Era*, Centre for the Study of Higher Education, Working Paper 87.14, Parkville: University of Melbourne.

Australian Universities Commission (1965) *Committee on the Future of Tertiary Education in Australia: Report* (The Martin Report), Canberra: Government Printer.

Ball, S.J. (1994) *Education Reform: A Critical and Poststructural Approach*, Buckingham: Open University Press.

Barry, A., Osborne, T. and Rose, N. (1996) *Foucault and Political Reason: Liberalism, Neo-liberalism and Rationalities of Government*, London: UCL Press.

Blair, T. (1997) 'Foreword', *Connecting the Learning Society*, London: HMSO. Online.
http://www.open.gov.uk/dfee/grid/foreword.htm.

Blair, T. (1998) 'Foreword', *The Learning Age: Towards a Europe of Knowledge*, European Union Conference, Lifelong Learning Conference, 17–19 May, Manchester, UK, London: HMSO. Online.
http://www.lifelonglearning.co.uk/conference/guide01.htm.

Blunkett, D. (1997) *Ministerial Statement: Higher Education*, House of Commons Hansard Debates, 23 July, columns 949–51.

Blunkett, D. (1998a) *The Learning Age: Towards a Europe of Knowledge*, European Union Conference, Lifelong Learning Conference, 17–19 May, Manchester: UK, London: HMSO. Online.
http://www.lifelonglearning.co.uk/conference/guide01.htm.

Blunkett, D. (1998b) *The Learning Age: A Renaissance for a New Britain*. Online.
http://www.lifelonglearning.co.uk/greenpaper/index.htm.

Brown, G. (1998) *Ministerial Statement: Comprehensive Funding Review*, House of Commons Hansard Debates, 14 July, (Part 5) column 190.

Brown, P. and Lauder, H. (1996) 'Education, globalisation and economic development', *Journal of Education Policy*, 11, 1: 1–26.

Burchell, G. (1991) 'Peculiar interests: civil society and governing "the system of natural liberty"', in G. Burchell, C. Gordon and P. Miller, *The Foucault Effect: Studies in Governmentality*, Hemel Hempstead, Herts.: Harverster Wheatsheaf.

Burchell, G. (1993) 'Liberal government and techniques of the self', *Economy and Society*, 22, 3: 267–82.

Burchell, G. (1996) 'Liberal government and techniques of the self', in A. Barry, T. Osborne and N. Rose (eds), *Foucault and Political Reason: Liberalismm Neo-liberalism and Rationalities of Government*, London: UCL Press.

Burchell, G., Gordon, C. and Miller, P. (1991) *The Foucault Effect: Studies in Governmentality*, Hemel Hempstead, Herts.: Harvester Wheatsheaf.

Cerny, P.G. (1990) *The Changing Architecture of Politics: Structure, Agency and the Future of the State*, London: Sage.

Commonwealth Tertiary Education Commission (Australia) (CTEC) (1986) *Review of Efficiency and Effectiveness in Higher Education*, Canberra: Australian Government Publishing Service.

Considine, M. (1988) 'The corporate management framework as administrative science: a critique', *Australian Journal of Public Administration*, 47, 1: 4–18.

Currie, J. and Newsome, J. (eds), (1998) *Universities and Globalization: Critical Perspectives*, Beverly Hills, CA: Sage.

Dawkins, J.S. (1983) *Reforming the Australian Public Service: A Statement of the Government's Intentions*, Canberra: Australian Government Publishing Service.

Dawkins, J.S. (1987) 'Minister's message', *DEET News*, 1, August.

Dawkins, J.S. (1988) *Higher Education: A Policy Statement*, Canberra: Australian Government Publishing Service.

Dawkins, J.S. and Holding, A.C. (1987) *Skills for Australia*, Canberra: Australian Government Publishing Service.

Dearing, R. (1997) *Higher Education in the Learning Society*, Report of the National Committee of Inquiry into Higher Education, London: HMSO. Online.
http://www.leeds.ac.uk/educol/ncihe/.

Dearing, R. (1998) 'The full-on university', *The Australian*, 14 October, 34–5.

The Discovering Democracy School Materials Project (1997) Carlton, Victoria: Curriculum Corporation.

Dudley, J. (1998) 'Globalization and education policy in Australia', in J. Currie and J. Newsome (eds), *Universities and Globalization: Critical Perspectives*, Beverly Hills, CA: Sage.

Education for Active Citizenship (1988) A Report by the Senate Standing Committee on Employment Education and Training, Canberra: Australian Government Publishing Service.

Emy, H.V. and Hughes, O.E. (1991) *Australian Politics: Realities in Conflict*, 2nd edn, South Melbourne: Macmillan.

Encouraging Citizenship (1990) House of Commons Commission on Citizenship, London: HMSO.

Further Education for the New Millennium (1988) London: HMSO. Online. http://www.lifelonglearning.co.uk/kennedy/index.htm.

Hawke, R.J. (1987) 'New machinery of government', the Prime Minister's media statement, 14 July, *Canberra Bulletin of Public Administration*, 52: 12–16.

Healy, G. and Richardson, J. (1998) 'Wary response to portfolio reshuffle', *The Australian*, 21 October: 37.

Higher Education for the 21st Century (1988) Response to the Dearing Report, London: HMSO. Online. http://www.lifelonglearning.co.uk/dearing/dr-fore.htm.

Illing, D. (1998) 'Postgraduates hold their edge', *The Australian*, 7 October: 28.

Kemp, D. (1998) *Strategic Developments in Higher Education*, Address to the OECD Thematic Review Seminar on the First Years of Tertiary Education, Sydney, 21 April.

The Learning Age: A Renaissance for a New Britain (1998) London: HMSO. Online. http://www.lifelonglearning.co.uk/greenpaper/index.htm.

The Learning Age: A Renaissance for a New Britain, A Summary (1998) London: HMSO. Online. http://www.lifelonglearning.co.uk/greenpaper/summary.pdf.

The Learning Age: Towards a Europe of Knowledge (1998) European Union Conference, Lifelong Learning Conference, 17–19 May, Manchester, UK, London: HMSO. Online. http://www.lifelonglearning.co.uk/conference/guide01.htm. http://www.lifelonglearning.co.uk/conference/guide02.htm.

Learning for the Twenty-first Century: First Report of the National Advisory Group for Continuing Education and Lifelong Learning (1997) London: HMSO. Online. http://www.lifelonglearning.co.uk/nagcell/index.htm.

Lingard, B., Knight, J. and Bartlett, L. (1993) *After the AEC: The Future of a National Agenda*, Australian Association for Research in Education Conference, Fremantle, Western Australia, 22 November.

Lingard, R. and Rizvi, F. (1998) 'Globalization, the OECD, and Australian higher education', in J. Currie and J. Newsome (eds), *Universities and Globalization: Critical Perspectives*, Beverly Hills, CA: Sage.

Marginson, S. (1993) *Education and Public Policy in Australia*, Melbourne: Cambridge University Press.

Marginson, S. (1997) *Educating Australia: Government, Economy and Citizen since 1960*, Melbourne: Cambridge University Press.

Marshall, N. (1988) 'Bureaucratic politics and the demise of the Commonwealth Tertiary Education Commission', *Australian Journal of Public Administration*, 47, 1: 19–34.

Meredyth, D. (1998) 'Corporatising education', in M. Dean and B. Hindess (eds), *Governing Australia: Studies in Contemporary Rationalities of Government*, Melbourne: Cambridge University Press, 20–46.

Moodie, G. (1998) 'Money will track teaching measures', *The Australian*, 7 October: 37.

Osmond, W. (1998) 'Kemp tightens education grip', *Campus Review*, 21–27 October: 1, 6.

Peters, M. (1996) *Poststructuralism, Politics, and Education*, Westport, CT: Bergin and Garvey.

Pusey, M. (1991) *Economic Rationalism in Canberra*, Melbourne: Cambridge University Press.

Report of the Committee on Australian Universities (The Murray Report) (1998) Canberra: Government Printer.

Review of Efficiency and Effectiveness in Higher Education (1986) Commonwealth Tertiary Education Commission, Canberra: Australian Government Publishing Service.

Rose, N. (1993) 'Government, authority and expertise in advanced liberalism', *Economy and Society*, 22, 3: 283–299.

Rose, N. (1996) 'Governing "advanced" liberal democracies', in A. Barry, T. Osborne and N. Rose (eds), *Foucault and Political Reason: Liberalism, Neo-liberalism and Rationalities of Government*, London: UCL Press.

Spencer, M. (1998) 'Surveys to measure return from education spending', *The Australian*, 7 October: 27.

Vidovich, L. and Porter, P. (1997) 'The recontextualisation of "quality" in Australian Higher Education', *Journal of Education Policy*, 12, 4: 233–52.

Walters, W. (1997) 'The "active society": new designs for social policy', *Policy and Politics*, 25, 3: 221–34.

West, R. (1998) *Learning for Life* (The West Review), Review of Higher Education Financing and Policy Review Committee, Canberra: Australian Government Publishing Service.

Whereas the People: Civics and Citizenship Education (1994) Report of the Civics Expert Group, Canberra: Australian Government Publishing Service.

Wran, N. (1998) *Report of the Committee on Higher Education Funding* (The Wran Report), Canberra: Australian Government Publishing Service.

Yeatman, A. (1990) *Bureaucrats, Technocrats, Femocrats*, Sydney: Allen and Unwin.

Question from Patricia: So, Janice, lifelong learning ... is it opportunity or sentence?

Response: Both – for whilst lifelong learning does provide the individual citizen with access to education and training throughout life (and hence, perhaps, protection against vulnerabilty and want in the uncertain world of the globalised economy) there is also the obligation, or requirement, for citizens to engage in retraining or reskilling throughout their working lives. Perhaps in a society in which there is provision against age discrimination and where compulsory retirement has been abolished, this sentence may be indeed lifelong – that is, for the term of one's natural life and ending only with death!

Learning for life – education and training – is directed principally towards the labour market and credentialism. Enhancing one's individual capacity to compete in the labour market necessarily enhances the nation's international capitalist competitiveness; and this is the contribution the citizen makes to the prosperity and security of the state. Of course, it should be acknowledged that in addition to enhancing the possibilities of greater personal economic security and prosperity, the opportunity to attain new credentials can be personally fulfilling. Learning for life, or the learning society, is certainly about self-development, self-betterment, in that it may provide the citizen with opportunities to undertake learning or education in areas of their life and experience beyond the simply economic. And I do believe that the model of choice around which the programmes are organised, rather than tutelage relationships of traditional welfare state (Yeatman 1994: 77) can be empowering.

Thus, learning for life does provide the opportunity to achieve self-development, self-actualisation. However, it is principally self-development in terms of the labour market. I think it's interesting to note that what is happening is that the language of emancipatory or liberatory humanism that has been/was characteristic of much education discourse, in for example the 1970s, has been coopted by post-Fordist 'responses' to the neo-liberal discourses of globalisation. In contrast to the present meaning of lifelong learning as enhancing labour market capacity, the emancipatory language of lifelong learning, or learning for life, is about self-actualisation, full development of the individual as a human being; in other words, becoming fully human. Self-development is an end in itself; the self is, in

Kantian terms, an end in its own right. The ethical rather than the economic is privileged, and education is a practice of freedom rather than of credentials.

Another dimension of lifelong learning as sentence is that, in what Ainley (1998) calls the 'certified society', there is an impoverished notion of what it is to learn. Learning is commodified. The learning which is valued is that which can be incorporated into capitalist economies, that which is marketable or saleable in the labour market. This necessarily limits the range of what can be learned – or what should be learned. Of course, knowledge is never neutral: any curriculum is necessarily selective and valorises some knowledges rather than others and is embedded within, and embeds particular relations of power and privilege. However, the discursive constitution of learning for life as principally economic does limit learning to the instrumental. Such objectives as openness to ideas, capacities for analysis and critical evaluative understanding, objectives which are characteristic of developmental or emancipatory education discourses are marginalised. Thus the citizen is sentenced not only to learning for the term of their natural lives, but also to a limited and impoverished range of learning experiences.

Learning for civic or altruistic participation in the life of the community is similarly marginalised. Although, for example, social inclusion and active citizenship constitute part of the language of lifelong learning, social inclusion is via individualistic contractual market relations rather than human interconnectedness. The learning society is a stakeholder society, where partnership forms the basis of social relations. Partnership is about particular forms of reciprocity – in Australia the language is of 'mutual obligation' as in the requirement that young people work for unemployment benefits (the pejoratively named 'Work for the Dole' scheme).

Thus the learning society is articulated with the reconstituting of welfare and the welfare state. However poorly realised, the postwar welfare model was a citizen's welfare state where benefits were the result of Marshallian social entitlement and all citizens were members by right. Citizenship, or membership of the imagined community, was membership of an ethical community based on political and moral equality. This membership afforded the citizen rights and obligations. However, in the post-welfare state (Ainley 1998: 566) – or the stakeholder society, or the learning society – the basis of social inclusion or membership is partnership, contribution and activity. Activity, such as learning, is one's social obligation to avert unemployment and hence welfare dependency. Welfare is a case of 'mutual obligation' and the recipient is required to demonstrate 'worthiness'. In the learning society 'worthiness' is to learn and to be prepared to learn for life. This is the contracting state (Harden in Ainley 1998: 563) in which contractual relations rather than citizenship entitlements organise social relations between citizens, and between citizens and the state. Social inclusion is predicated on the citizen, or welfare or education recipient, being 'account-able for fulfilling the conditions of the contract' (Ainley 1998: 567). The conditions of the contract are partnership, mutual obligation, activity and contribution, whilst the earlier concept of entitlement – either in terms of Marshall's social rights or as a Kantian ethical entity in one's own right – is reconstituted as welfare dependency.

The contractual obligation of the citizen is open ended – that is, life-long. In the learning society, learning is for life; in other words, to learn, to reskill, to retrain is an obligation that can never be fully met. The conditions of this unequal contract are such that it can never be concluded.

The policies of the learning society constitute a series of normalising practices where the good and responsible citizen is the individual who learns and continues to learn. It is to such a citizen that the stakeholder society owes an obligation. However, the 'citizen' who either does not or refuses to learn is irresponsible and 'bad'. By implication, to such an individual the society owes little. However, it is not an inhumane society: there is a safety net for those who, for reasons beyond their control, are unable to participate fully as active partners in social life. However, for both the 'bad' and the 'incapable' citizen, full and equal participation in the life of the community – the fundamental of social inclusion or citizenship – is a chimera.

I think these themes are particularly well illustrated by the 1998 European Union Conference, *The Learning Age: Towards a Europe of Knowledge* (http://www.lifelonglearning.co.uk/conference/guide01.htm):

> We are in a new age – the age of information and of global com-petition. Familiar certainties and old ways of doing things are disappearing. The types of jobs we do have changed as have the industries in which we work and the skills they need. At the same time opportunities are opening up as we see the potential of new technologies to change our lives for the better.

> In the Learning Age we will need a workplace with the skills, im-agination and confidence to see us into the new century.

Many thousands of occupations demand different types of knowledge and understanding and the skills to apply them. That is what we mean by skills, and it is through learning – with the help of those who teach us – that we acquire them.

Learning's contribution to community development and social inclusion, to fostering a sense of citizenship, responsibility and identity is as important as its contribution to the economy. We must strive to bridge 'the learning divide' – between those who have benefited from education and training and those who have not.

The capacity to cope with change will be the hallmark of success in the twenty-first century ...

...

... Towards a Europe of Knowledge

Economic competitiveness, employment and the personal fulfilment of the citizens of Europe is no longer mainly based on the production of physical goods, nor will it be in the future. Real wealth creation will henceforth be linked to the production and dissemination of knowledge and will depend first and foremost on our efforts in the field of research, education and training and on our capacity to promote innovation. This is why we must fashion a true 'Europe of Knowledge'.

This process is directly linked to the aim of developing lifelong learning which the Union has set itself and which has been incorporated into the Amsterdam Treaty, expressing the determination of the Union to *promote the highest level of knowledge for its people through broad access to education and its permanent updating.*

(Original emphasis)

References

Ainley, P. (1998) 'Towards a learning or a certified society? Contradictions in the New Labour modernization of lifelong learning', *Journal of Education Policy*, 13, 4: 559–73.

The Learning Age: Towards a Europe of Knowledge (1998), European Union Conference, Lifelong Learning Conference, 17–19 May, Manchester, UK. http://www.lifelonglearning.co.uk/conference/guide01.htm

Yeatman, A. (1994) *Postmodern Revisionings of the Political*, London: Routledge.

Question from Ian: Universities have always been regarded as key institutions in civil society and, if you like, schools for citizenship. How do you think the reconstruction of academic life in terms of neo-liberalism has affected this civic character of academic practice, both in terms of the identities and practices of academics and the nature of university teaching? As a university researcher and teacher yourself, what sort of tensions do you experience (if any!) between older civic or social democratic university discourses and practices and those of our contemporary corporatising academy?

Response: Certainly, Ian, academic life and hence our practice, and also our sense of self as academics, are being reshaped fundamentally by the neo-liberal 'imperatives' governing universities. I think your term 'our contemporary corporatising academy' is a neat summary of what is happening in universities at present. I like particularly that you do not appear to assume that it's all over – as evidenced by your use of the term *corporatising* (present tense) rather than *corporatised* (past tense). You do therefore seem to be saying that there are possibilities for 'resisting' this 'corporatising'. I'll return to this possibility later.

In my chapter I didn't talk much about the managerialism dominating universities at present, but it's an element of the neo-liberal reform agenda. Basic to the microeconomic reform of universities themselves is the introduction and continuing development of managerialist practice comparable to that of the corporate world. A model of managerialism is the basis in the reform documents, such as the Dawkins White Paper of 1988 and the later Hoare Review (1995) in Australia and the Dearing Review (1997) in Britain, which show a concern with the size of institutions' governing bodies and their resemblance to the boards of directors of corporations. Similarly it underpins the reconstitution of the role of Vice-Chancellor as Chief Executive Officer – even on occasion the VC being 'rebadged' as CEO.

I think you'd agree that we should be wary of idealising the past as some golden age. Universities were traditionally elite institutions to which access had been limited, principally to those from more privileged backgrounds. In addition, they were – and are – patriarchal places, both for students and staff (Burton 1997). Traditional practice was based on discourses of common culture and heritage with the commensurate incapacities and resistances to acknowledging or dealing with difference and heterogeneity. The curriculum itself was gendered and culturally oppressive, reinforcing, if not reproducing, social disadvantage and capitalist social relations.

However, whilst acknowledging their faults, I agree with you regarding the civic character of university teaching and learning. The so-called 'liberal values' (not to be confused with the neo-liberalism of the last decades), that is the values of tolerance, critical enquiry, openness to ideas, breadth of learning and learning 'for its own sake' rather than narrowly vocational training, have been central to what universities have offered to their societies. And in the 1970s many institutions offered and attempted to manifest values which could best be summarised as 'emancipatory humanism'. Ball (1998: 191) refers to 'metaphysical discourses around social justice and equality ... fables of promise and opportunity'.

It is the universities' intellectual traditions and ideals that are under challenge, if not threat, from neo-liberal discourses of globalisation and the 'imperatives' that flow from the 'inevitability' of global economic integration. These intellectual traditions have included academic freedom, a culture of critical engagement with society, the search for 'truth', 'pure' research and the pursuit of knowledge for its own sake. Organisational traditions included institutional autonomy and collective, collegial decision making. The social contribution made by the academy was assumed, recognised and affirmed. Of course I'd again emphasise that these traditions are idealised and that there are both positive and negative elements to each of them. I'd also emphasise that, whilst university autonomy and academic freedom are discursive, so too emancipatory humanism and the traditions which link the modern academy to the medieval foundations are themselves metanarratives.

In contrast to these traditions, the current practices of academics are being governed by performance indicators, guidelines, templates, evaluation and accountability requirements. Professionalism and autonomy are being replaced by 'perpetual scrutiny' (Rose in Marginson 1997: 167). Managerialist practices exclude academics from substantive decision making as important decisions are made by managers rather than by academics, whilst academics are increasingly required to carry out the decisions made elsewhere – at Vice-Chancellorial level or Pro-Vice-Chancellorial level or by executive deans. This is 'steering at a distance' with academics having little role in establishing policy decisions yet being required to implement them.

In terms of the changing character of university teaching, there is a growing instrumentalism, especially with respect to students. Rather than students being considered as ends in their own right, they are increasingly being commodified – especially with the growth in full-fee courses at postgraduate level. A parallel commodification of the students' learning itself is produced by the additional cost pressures on students – fees and user-pays practices within universities, together with the decline in adequate financial support from society, as manifested in grants (UK) or support schemes such as Austudy (Australia). In addition, higher workloads and pressures to 'do more with less' challenge academics' professional commitments to quality teaching.

Self-surveillance, self-evaluation and self-improvement in terms of externally imposed criteria constitute professional development. In other words, professional development is being reconfigured to constitute adhering to or mastering management priorities more effectively. Academics are as Willmott's employees, 'simultaneously required, individually and collectively, to recognise and *take responsibility for* the relationship between the security of their employment and their contribution to the competitiveness of the goods and services they produce' (Ball 1998: 193; emphasis in original). This is the 'new professionalism' (ibid.: 195).

Our colleague, Jan Currie from Murdoch's School of Education, is engaged in a long-term study, 'The Changing Nature of Academic Work' (Currie and Vidovich 1998; Vidovich and Currie 1998). The results of Jan's project demonstrate that increased accountability requirements are a key feature of the changing nature of academic work, together with a decreased sense of autonomy with respect to work (Vidovich et *al.* 1996a, 1996b). Academics report a general sense of disillusionment and demoralisation (Pears et *al.* 1996), and a loss of a sense of control over their professional practice. Many report health problems such as sleep disturbance, increased levels of infection, ill health, general malaise and diminished feelings of well-being (Currie et *al.* 1996).

There is also a loss of societal recognition of the worth of academic work: through the declining real value of salaries and status, but perhaps more importantly through the lack of affirmation reflected back to academics by the society they serve by the media, by some but not all students, but most particularly by governments (Pears et *al.* 1996).

Ball (1990: 156) refers to management as a technology of power, a regime of truth, and certainly managerialist practices are disempowering.

Managerialism constitutes a deprofessionalising, effectively a deskilling, of academic work and hence is experienced as an attack on their identities or subjectivities by academics themselves. The stress of value tension is intellectually enervating:

> [T]he [academic's] commitments, sense of professional identity, sense of self and self worth are beset by tensions and contradictions. An old and a new subjectivity vie with one another, producing another kind of personal incoherence and dissonance – a fragmentation of the self. The 'nostalgia for the lost narrative' conflicts with new forms of legitimation.
>
> (Ball 1998: 195)

Finally, you ask what sort of tensions are experienced between older civic or social democratic university discourses and practices and those of our contemporary corporatising academy?

There is certainly some loss of a sense of community, whilst competition between departments and schools is heightened – principally as a manifestation of the internal politics of scarcity over distribution of funding within institutions rather than as intellectual disputation. There is a need to 'sell' oneself and one's work and the work of one's department. We resort to 'image' and the languages of advertising, but these do not sit well with the traditions and rigour of peer review. Even those in 'successful' departments or 'popular' disciplines feel disquiet at the ruthless marginalising, or excision, of 'non-economic' disciplines and fields of study, or the need for such disciplines to argue their relevance in econometric language. We see evidence that institutions are reverting to the elitism and patriarchalism of the past, whilst intellectual traditions that are highly valued – such as academic freedom – are threatened (see, for example, Kelsey 1998).

Certainly as individuals we are either becoming more pragmatic and instrumental, or the contradictions and dilemmas are causing considerable anger or heartache and despair. However, I don't want to give the impression that 'resistance' is useless. And I'll talk about this in terms of the personal and the strategic.

First, the capacity to analyse university policies and practices and their discursive character cannot only provide insights, but can also enable one as an individual to be – or at least feel – less tossed and battered as though by unexpected and unknown storms. For some, this opens opportunities for the subversion, or at least the reconfiguration, of the guidelines that we are required to work within. Moreover, the capacity to analyse the discursive character of events and policies, together with a sense of contingency that comes from the postmodern relieves one of the need for a sense of absolute control, and hence is in itself a new form of control over one's destiny.

At the strategic level, many academics are attempting to accommodate the instrumental requirements of the new context without compromising that which they believe to be of value from the past, whilst others attempt to subvert neo-liberal practices; so that, for example, even if equity is constituted as maximising the nation's human capital, in one's own practice it can be effected in terms of Ball's (1988: 191) 'metaphysical discourses around social justice and equality'.

I would argue, also, that there is the need to take advantage of the fact that some of the language of accountability can be turned to advantage – accountability is not necessarily, and only, financial. Accountability is also about democracy and citizenship. Indeed, in a democratic society, it can be argued to be of considerably greater significance than any mere financial balancing of the books. To insist, for example, on the language of collective democratic accountability and its commensurate need for transparency and openness; to insist on the need for democratic practice in institutional governance – for example, to resist the model of governing bodies being based upon boards of directors of corporations; to insist on students and staff being considered as citizens of the institution and thus able to draw upon the citizenship languages of the ethical community, of ethical and political equality, and of universalism, are strategies that counter the totalising discourses of economism and international competitiveness. These contrasting languages of accountability are expressive of the tension between the competing discursive fundamentals of democracy and capitalism, the set of contradictions which is inevitably embedded in liberal democratic capitalist societies.

I could go on almost indefinitely about this, Ian! However, I'll finish by saying that this discussion – of the intersections between one's personal ideals with respect to teaching and research, and one's personal subjectivity as an academic, with both university policies and practices and also the wider context of neo-liberal governance – has been an instance of reflective practice. In my view, it is through reflective practice that alternative discursive possibilities can become apparent.

References

Ball, S.J. (1990) 'Management as moral technology: a Luddite analysis', in S.J. Ball (ed.) *Foucault and Education: Disciplines and Knowledge*, London: Routledge, 153–166.

Ball, S.J. (1998) 'Performativity and fragmentation in "postmodern schooling"', in John Carter (ed.) *Postmodernity and the Fragmentation of Welfare*, London: Routledge, 18–203.

Burton, C. (1997) with the editorial assistance of Linda Cook and Susan Wilson, *Gender Equity in Australian University Staffing*, Canberra: Department of Employment, Education, Training and Youth Affairs.

Currie, J., Vidovich, L., Welch, A. and Pears, H. (1996) 'Trends report on stress and morale', in *The Changing Nature of Academic Work: Case Study of Murdoch University, March 1996*, unpublished paper, Murdoch University and Sydney University.

Currie, J., Vidovich, L. and H. Pears (1996) 'Trends report on sense of community at Murdoch University', *The Changing Nature of Academic Work: Case Study of Murdoch University, June 1996*, unpublished paper, School of Education, Murdoch University.

Currie, J. and Vidovich, L. (1998) 'Microeconomic reform through managerialism in American and Australian universities', in Jan Currie and Janice Newsome (eds), *Universities and Globalization: Critical Perspectives*, Beverly Hills, CA: Sage.

Dawkins, J.S. (1988) *Higher Education: A Policy Statement*, Canberra: Australian Government Publishing Service.

Dearing, R. (1997) *Higher Education in the Learning Society*, Report of the National Committee of Inquiry into Higher Education, London: HMSO. Online. http://www.leeds.ac.uk/niche/natrep.htm.

Hoare, D. (1995) *Report of the Committee of Inquiry*, Higher Education Management Review Committee, Canberra: Australian Government Publishing Service.

Kelsey, J. (1998) *Academic Freedom: Needed Now More Than Ever*. Online. http: /webnz.com.aus/papers/acfreed.htm.

Marginson, S. (1997) *Educating Australia: Government, Economy and Citizen since 1960*, Melbourne: Cambridge University Press.

Pears, H., Currie, J. and Vidovich, L. (1996) 'Trends report on the importance of work in the lives of academics', in *The Changing Nature of Academic Work: Case Study of Murdoch University, August 1996*, unpublished paper, School of Education, Murdoch University.

Vidovich, L., Currie, J. and Pears, H. (1996a) 'Trends report on accountability and autonomy', in *The Changing Nature of Academic Work: Case Study of Murdoch University, August 1996*, unpublished paper, School of Education, Murdoch University.

Vidovich, L., Currie, J. and Pears, H. (1996b) 'Trends report on decision making styles', in *The Changing Nature of Academic Work: Case Study of Murdoch University, October 1996*, unpublished paper, School of Education, Murdoch University.

Vidovich, L. and Currie, J. (1998) 'Changing accountability and autonomy at the "coalface" of academic work in Australia', in Jan Currie and Janice Newsome (eds), *Universities and Globalization: Critical Perspectives*, Beverly Hills, CA: Sage, 193–212.

Question from Alan: Many of those on the Left have critiqued the emergence of the corporatist ethos in universities on the grounds that it undermines pedagogic and scholarly ideals; e.g. the spirit of enquiry and collegiality. However, universities have traditionally been sites for the production of privileged knowledges and for upholding privileged statuses, particularly those based on socioeconomic status and differences of gender, sexuality and ethnicity. How can poststructuralism help us rethink the relationship between the higher education system and social inequality? To what extent and in what ways does poststructuralism challenge assumptions held by Marxists and an earlier generation of feminists about the nature of this relationship?

Response: Alan, as I think I acknowledged in my response to Ian, I'd agree that universities have 'traditionally been sites for the production of privileged knowledges and for upholding privileged statuses, particularly those based on socioeconomic status and differences of gender, sexuality and ethnicity'. However, I believe that they have been places of collegiality and enquiry also. They have been both – and more. In other words, universities, like any other complex social institution, are not uni-discursive sites. Rather, they are multi-discursive, with the tensions and contradictions necessarily generated by variously competing, complementary and conflicting discourses.

You've asked me how poststructuralism can help us to rethink the relationship between the higher education system and social inequality. Poststructuralist analysis focuses on the minutiae, or the detail, of daily routines and also of the policies and practices which regulate our behaviours, our interactions with colleagues and students and our teaching practices. Therefore, such an approach enables us to analyse the manner in which the minutiae of daily practice work either to maintain existing or establish new forms of unequal power relations, and hence social inequality

– whether based on gender, socio-economic status, ethnicity, race or sexuality. In my chapter I've demonstrated that the principles of neo-liberal thought and neo-classical economics are organising and structuring higher education policy. And, of course, the intent of policy is to structure and organise practice. Therefore to analyse the discursive principles underlying the policies which are intended to shape and structure practice enables a poststructuralist analysis to explore the practices which manifest and structure the relationship between higher education and inequality.

The neo-classical liberalism which is the organising principle of higher education policy and management practices is intended to delimit and structure our behaviours, our interactions with colleagues and students and our teaching practices in accordance with the discursive 'truths' of economic rationalism/neo-liberalism. These require, for example, that university practices be grounded on assumptions of competitive individualism, of the privileging of the public over the private, of the privileging of the economic over the social more broadly – in other words, that a human being is economic man or *homo economicus* rather than a social entity with the potential for altruisism. Economic rationalism, or neo-classical liberalism, is the quintessential discourse of late twentieth-century modernity: instrumental and patriarchal, valorising the economic and subjugating the non-human natural world.

It is important to be clear that whilst the discourses of economic rationalism or neo-liberalism are elitist, they are not overtly discriminatory – there is a strong equity focus in recent higher education policies, indeed education policies more broadly, although it is equity in terms of human capital rather than in terms of individual self-determination. Neither neo-liberalism nor neo-classical economics is concerned with social inequality except in so far as all have equal formal status as parties to contract(s). Issues of the equality or inequality of material circumstances are simply not relevant, as they are assumed to be the outcome of competitive behaviour between equally empowered individuals.

However, many of the policies and practices now taken for granted in universities – such as user pays – are likely to affect the material circumstances of individuals differently. Clearly, those of lower socioeconomic status have less capacity to pay and hence participate, whilst the strong correlations between economic capacity and gender, race and ethnicity – whilst complex – are empirically demonstrable. Hence the assumption within neo-liberal economically rational policies of the sovereign, equally empowered individual necessarily advantages those from backgrounds of higher socioeconomic or otherwise material circumstances. Such polices and hence much of the day-to-day practice of higher education therefore re-embed or maintain existing social and power relations.

If power is 'the structuring of the possible field of action by others' (Peters 1996: 82), that is structuring the potential for agency or life choices of individuals, then neo-liberal, economically rational discourses limit the potential for agency, differentially in terms of the individual's social positioning with respect to gender, ethnicity, race and class. In other words, economically rational or neo-liberal policies empower individuals differentially in terms of their social positioning with respect to gender, ethnicity, race and class.

Whereas Marxists might claim that material inequality is derived from structures of power determined by the economic structure of society and, hence, that economic relations determine power relations between individuals and groups, the claim of neo-liberal, neo-classical economic models or economic rationalism is that economic and/or social inequality is the inevitable outcome of rational individualistic self-interested utility-maximising behaviour. Poststructuralism analyses material inequality and inequalities of power as the results of discursive practices which valorise particular forms of behaviour, policies and practices. Subjectivity is similarly discursively constituted and, in turn, particular forms of subjectivity lead to behaviours, policies and practices which result in inequality either of material circumstances and/or power.

In my view, whilst poststructuralism is analytical rather than normative, that does not mean that poststructuralists cannot engage with ethical issues. Poststructuralism does, after all, come from a critical tradition. Thus, for example, a poststructuralist perspective does not deny the common good; rather, to acknowledge that 'the common good' is discursively constituted problematises, or opens up, such ethical or normative issues for contest and debate.

That there are no certainties, no absolutes, no fundamental truths, but rather, as Patricia said in her response to your question, 'conditions of possibility' underlying current truths, opens the future to human agency. If indeed power is structuring the field of agency, agency is central – in terms of concrete material circumstances and practices, at the level of individual practice and departmental priorities, and also at senior administrative and policy levels.

Finally, if unchallenged, the policies and practices of the new academy, in what is variously referred to as the post welfare state, the competition state, the post-Fordist state and the contracting state, are likely to maintain or worsen existing unequal social and power relationships, or alternatively create new forms of inequality. However, similarly to the traditional university, the new academy is not uni-discursive. Coexisting both comfortably and uncomfortably are the totalising regime of truth that is neo-liberal, neo-classical economics and older and/or alternative discourses. These include not only the traditional discriminatory regimes of patriarchy, ethnocentricity, sexual and gender discrimination, and racial discrimination, but also ideals of education as social, human centred and emancipatory.

There is no certainty. The future is 'up for grabs'.

Reference

Peters, M. (1996) *Poststructuralism, Politics and Education*, Westport, CT: Bergin and Garvey.

Chapter 4

Public health, the new genetics and subjectivity

Alan Petersen

This chapter examines how the new genetics is shaping our ways of thinking about and responding to problems in public health and explores some implications of this development for how we conceptualise policy. Genetic knowledge is rapidly finding applications in public health, isolating new objects of analysis and delineating new areas of intervention. Genomics is being rapidly assimilated into technologies of screening and prenatal diagnosis and in practices of counselling and is likely to find future applications in genetic therapies. While there has been much discussion in the scientific literature and in the media about both the potential health benefits and the ethical dilemmas and dangers of this development, there has been little analysis of its underlying rationalities and of how these shape subjectivity and action. Genetics is radically altering the way we view our bodies, conduct ourselves and interact with others. In this chapter, I examine how genetic knowledge is helping to redefine the natural and the normal, and hence our concepts of the body and disease, our perceptions of appropriate treatment and prevention, and views of responsible citizenship. I also explore the possibilities created by this development for contesting the imperatives of health and the meanings of citizenship. In raising and exploring these questions, I have been strongly influenced by the governmentality literature. Governmentality scholars have focused on the processes of rule in contemporary societies, examining in particular how we govern ourselves as particular kinds of subjects. These questions have been largely neglected in both the 'mainstream' and critical public health literature, but are ones which, I believe, need to become more central in analyses of public health policy.

In public health, as in other areas of policy, there has been a tendency to take the aims and objects of policy as relatively unproblematic givens. Although there is a relatively long tradition in policy studies in which it is recognised that policy 'constructs' its problems, policy is viewed, by and large, as a reaction to real, objective conditions. Thus, public health has been defined as a multidisciplinary field of research and action, involving 'the epidemiological study of the health conditions of populations', and 'the study of the organized social response to those conditions, in particular, the way in which such response is structured through the health care system' (Frenk 1993: 472). This and other similar definitions reflect what Osborne (1997) refers to as a reactive conception of the relationship between policy and its objects. In public health, policy is seen as a reaction to objective problems of health need and provision, and the state of health is seen as a reflection of the effectiveness of policy (ibid.: 173). As Osborne notes, even the so-called critical approaches to health policy, which introduce a historical dimension into their analyses and focus on clashes of interest between different parties or interest groups, tend to adopt a reactive conception of policy in so far as they are concerned with measuring the distance between the provision of policy and objectively existing conditions. The most notable examples are Marxist histories of health policies which, as Osborne explains, see policy as the (unusually inadequate) outcome of the negotiations between different interest groups resulting from some agreed intolerable situation. The point that tends to be overlooked by those who adopt this conception of policy, but has been emphasised by governmentality scholars, is that the objects of policies are always products of particular problematisations. In other words, far from being reactive, policy is highly productive: it constitutes certain fields for action or inaction, and brings into play a specific array of social regulations. To define a problem in a particular way (e.g. as a product of the environment or of biological make-up) presupposes the invocation of certain strategies and practices and the existence of particular kinds of selves and subjectivities. In order to appreciate properly what is unique about the rationalities that are associated with contemporary, genetics-based public health, I believe it is important first to understand the broader shifts in conceptions of society that have been discernible within the discourses of public health.

Broad shifts in conceptions of society within discourses of public health

For much of the last two hundred years, public health discourse, like many other areas of social thought, has been underpinned by two major understandings of society: one which focuses on its law-like character; the other which centres on its historical nature and the historical constitution of knowledge and the application of knowledge to improve society. As Rabinow (1989: 24) explains: 'the sciences of man in the nineteenth and twentieth centuries are a litany of attempts to perfect one or the other of these approaches, or to combine them in a grander synthesis'. In the first conception, society is seen as an aspect of the natural world, comprising functionally interrelated parts and governed by underlying law-like universal mechanisms. This conception employs the so-called organic metaphor, whereby society is seen to have its own dynamic, and is described as having its own health and pathologies, the norms for which can be objectively known. This conception was evident in nineteenth-century concerns about the 'diseases of civilisation': the notion that the social body itself was sick. Tuberculosis, for instance, was seen as a classic disease of civilisation and its incidence was clearly associated with the big city's unwholesome environment: damp, smoke, overcrowding.

In the second conception, humans are able to utilise knowledge for self-understanding and to perfect society. Thus, it is believed that scientific understanding of society and of the pattern of disease causation can be applied for the improvement of individual bodies and of the social body as a whole. Public health proponents frequently look back to nineteenth-century public health as an example of how rational knowledge combined with rational administration can lead to improved living and working conditions for the mass of the population. Policy is seen as an instrument of social betterment, used for ameliorating the pathologies which threaten to disrupt the harmony of the organic whole. Elements of both these views of society are evident in many histories of public health; that is, the focus on epidemics (which are viewed as law-like in their development and manifestation), great scientific discoveries (i.e. learning how the organism 'works') and sanitary reforms (the reflexive application of new knowledge for social betterment). Very often, the development of public health policy is portrayed as an outcome of a gradual awakening, involving increasing recognition of the objective environmental conditions affecting health, the struggle for reform by a group of gallant individuals, and growing appreciation of the need for rational (i.e. scientific) understanding and concerted governmental action. The sanitary reformers frequently appear as heroes who laid the groundwork for a 'public health movement' and who were largely responsible for bringing about the improvements in the living and working conditions now enjoyed by the bulk of the population, or at least those residing in the rich western world.

According to governmentality scholars, these conceptions of society began to emerge during the late eighteenth century and the nineteenth century with the beginnings of concerns about how to correctly govern the population. As Foucault pointed out, although an explicit and intense interest in the art of government – how to govern others, how to be governed, by whom people will accept being governed, how to become the best governor, and so on – was evident in Europe much earlier (in the sixteenth century), in the eighteenth century population became the central theme and 'ultimate end of government' (Foucault 1991: 100–1). Concerns about the health, happiness and well-being of the population were expressed through the concept of police, defined as 'the science of happiness' or 'the science of government' (Pasquino 1991: 108). New forms of knowledge and new ways of acting in relation to the population emerged during this period, creating new sub-divisions by age, sex, and occupation, 'posing their different problems which require different sorts of intervention, a population which no longer merely lives and dies, but has a birth rate and death rate' (ibid. 1991: 115).

In Rosen's view, interest in health as a question of public policy gained prominence through the concept of medical police in the third quarter of the eighteenth century, but was superseded by terms such as 'public health' and 'hygiene' in the last quarter of the nineteenth century (Rosen 1974: 134, 153). Medical police focused on the practical conditions of security, with supervising the health of the population in order to produce healthy subjects who would be able to fulfil their obligations in peace and war. It involved the creation of a medical policy by government and its implementation through administrative regulation. There was a growing concern to regulate medical education, supervise apothecary shops and hospitals, prevent epidemics, combat quackery and enlighten the public (ibid.: 138). Rosen has described the consolidation of a socially orientated view of health and disease in the nineteenth century which focused on the concept of the social group, and more specifically social class. The idea of medicine as a social science gained increasing credibility during the nineteenth century leading eventually to clarification of the concept of social medicine. The growing awareness of the relationship of medicine to social problems was reflected in Virchow's famous slogan: 'Medicine is a social science, and politics is nothing but medicine on a grand scale' (ibid.: 62).

The use of statistics to analyse public health problems from the 1820s onwards reflected the consolidation of the scientific understanding of society as an entity governed by norms and probabilities (Hacking 1990). Statistics constructed an ideal, objective state for health, and allowed distinctions to be drawn between the normal and the pathological. According to Rabinow (1989: 67), the emergence of statistics signalled that society had at last become an object to be understood and reformed, and that the normality and pathology of the individual was seen as a function not of the individual's independent moral state but of his or her place within the whole. Statistics were used to measure the incidence of different diseases and to compare social groups and changes over time, providing the basis for a risk assessment of socially objective causes. Statistical data on social and environmental conditions were referred to extensively in the reports of the Poor Law Commission, established in 1834, as well as in Chadwick's classic *Report on the Sanitary Condition of the Labouring Population of Great Britain* (1842), and in the report of the Health of Towns Commission (1844). In Chadwick's report, for example, one can find detailed statistics on birth rates (e.g. ratio of births to the whole population in different locations, proportion of illegitimate births to total births), death rates (e.g. ages of death, causes of death, years lost by premature death), and the 'comparative chance of life in different classes' (measured by the proportion of deaths in different age cohorts for different occupational groups) (Flinn 1965). Such statistical calculations have been premised upon the post-Enlightenment modernist ideal that through rational counting and ordering problems could be brought under control (Hacking 1990: 3). As Bauman (1997: 11) has argued, such statistical 'order-making' has been integral to efforts within modern societies to draw lines between the pure and the impure, and to cleanse that which is seen to be 'foreign'. The process of defining the norm, and measuring deviations from that norm, implies the existence of the abnormal which should be reformed, controlled or eliminated. In the past, the drawing of the *cordon sanitaire* was a physical means of excluding the other, or keeping a separation between the 'clean' and the 'dirty'. This has typically involved restricting the movements of whole populations, including keeping some groups locked up or under constant surveillance through ongoing physical observation.

Although these views of society are still pervasive, they have gradually been eroded and, more and more, we are seeing conceptions of society based on the rationality of 'the market' and the notion of the individual as sovereign citizen. As Nikolas Rose (1994: 46) puts it: ' "society" (the sum of the bonds and relations between individuals and events which is governed by its own laws) as invented by social scientists of the nineteenth century, has begun to lose its self-evidence as a mechanism for governing people by acting upon social bonds'. In its place, there has emerged a new 'rationality of rule' – a way of thinking about and acting upon problems – which has been variously called 'advanced liberalism', or 'neo-liberalism', the features of which have been extensively described elsewhere (see, e.g., Rose and Miller 1992; Rose 1996). With neo-liberal rule, the emphasis is on the entrepreneurial subject and on generating conditions that will facilitate autonomous, self-directed action. The question of how individuals think and feel and of how to create environments supportive of 'psychosocial well-being' are now of concern to public health authorities. Like older discourses of public health, contemporary public health has its experts, who continue to play a crucial role as advisers, who collect and analyse information (particularly of a statistical nature), define appropriate norms and come up with appropriate solutions. However, expertise is of a greater variety and is located in diverse public and private spheres, and individuals are now called upon to play an active role in resolving their own problems and in seeking out appropriate expertise. It is in this context that the notions of active citizenship and citizen participation have come to the fore.

Active citizenship is frequently invoked as a defence against governmental or bureaucratic intrusion and is contrasted with earlier 'top-down', paternalistic forms of intervention that are seen as characteristic of the period of sanitary reform (see, e.g., Ashton and Seymour 1988; Bracht and Tsouros 1990; Pike *et al.* 1990; Bracht 1991). Many public health experts define their role in terms of facilitating the process of democratisation, or of 'enabling' or 'empowering' individuals and groups (e.g. Wallerstein 1993; Yeo 1993). They see themselves as mediators, overcoming the 'barriers' to 'participation' through increasing levels of awareness about the determinants of health, helping individuals to use the media in an effective way, lobbying politicians, and encouraging citizens to adopt a more 'health-conscious' approach to life. From the governmentality perspective, active citizenship is seen as one of the key mechanisms by which subjects come to exercise a regulated freedom under neo-liberal rule. To emphasize *regulated* freedom is not to deny human agency, for this is fundamental to neo-liberal techniques of government, but rather to recognise that the forms of action that are seen to constitute autonomous ('free') action are constrained and closely aligned with official objectives (see Garland 1997: 196–7).

From eugenics to the new genetics

These broad shifts have been reflected in discourses of heredity that have emerged during the twentieth century. Ideas about society as having a law-like character, as being perfectible and as subject to rational management were prominent in early twentieth-century thinking about heredity and efforts to improve populations through selective breeding, that is eugenics. Eugenics arose in a context of concerns about the degeneration of civilisation, resulting in particular from the mixing of the 'races', and aimed to put the 'hereditary flow' in order by eliminating the 'unhealthy' and undesirable and blocking the reproduction of inferior blood (Grau 1995: 4). According to the eugenicists, the sociopolitical arrangements (the tax system, the Poor Laws, indiscriminate charity) were encouraging the unfit to breed and dissuading better and more-responsible stock from self-perpetuation. Some groups (e.g. gypsies) were judged as 'throw-backs' who were unable to cope with modernity and progress, and therefore needed 'a helping hand towards inevitable extinction' (Porter 1993: 594–5). The term 'racial hygiene' adopted by some writers during the period of eugenics neatly captures the concern to preserve the purity of white European stock from contamination by 'impure' others. Eugenics was based upon the following premises (see Allen 1996: 24):

- a firm trust in the methods of selective breeding as a means of improving the quality of the human species;
- a belief in the power of heredity to directly determine physical, physiological and mental (including personality) traits in adults;

- an inherent belief in the inferiority of some races and the superiority of others, but including ethnic groups and social classes as well;
- a faith in the power of rational science to solve social problems, including those seen as intractable such as urban and labour violence, and to eliminate various forms of mental disease, including manic depression, schizophrenia and feeble-mindedness.

The doctrine of scientific management, involving trained experts in the setting of economic and social objectives, and the identification and prevention of problems before they occur in the name of efficiency, was part of the progressive ideology in many societies, including the United States, Germany, England, France, Italy and Scandinavia, in the early twentieth century. However, as Allen points out, most work occurred in Germany and the United States and grew from a common economic and social experience, involving boom-and-bust economic cycles, periods of raging inflation, rising unemployment, declining rates of profit and labour unrest. In both Europe and the United States, the response to these conditions by the economically and politically powerful was to attempt to bring a *laissez-faire* economy (involving little government interference) and associated political and social practices under control. Eugenics was seen as a scientific means of managing population in order to protect the biological quality of the local stock and to make society more efficient, particularly by halting the rise of 'defective' immigrants and preventing the biologically degenerate and unfit from reproducing. Towards this end, in the 1920s and 1930s, eugenical sterilisation laws were passed in 30 states in the US and in Nazi Germany (Allen 1996: 24–8; Kevles 1995: 93–4, 107–111, 116–17).

Some writers see clear parallels between the conditions that gave rise to eugenics and those giving rise to the new genetics; namely, a declining economic situation, involving falling weekly earnings, growing disparities in wealth and high levels of unemployment. As Allen observes, as in the Weimar and Nazi periods in Germany, in the United States today (and, one could add, elsewhere) there have been debates about who should receive what kind of health care and for how long: 'In the "cutback" atmosphere that dominates our discussions of other social policies, the mood seems similarly exclusionary and bitter' (Allen 1996: 29–30). Concerns about the use of new genetic knowledge for 'selective breeding', particularly through the routine use of prenatal genetic diagnosis, has led some commentators to warn of the dangers of a revived eugenics, or a neo-eugenics, movement. However, in contemporary liberal democratic societies, the explicit articulation of such ideas is, by and large, unacceptable and in some societies (particularly in Europe) concern about such an eventuality has given rise to new ethical guidelines and legislation. Thus the operation of a eugenic law in China, which compels all couples to undergo testing before marriage for mental disorders, sexually transmitted diseases and 'serious hereditary diseases' and, if found to suffer from a disease, submit to sterilisation or abortion, or remain celebate in order to prevent 'inferior births', is considered repugnant in many western liberal democracies (Dikötter 1998).

The discursive link between 'risk' and responsibility

In noting these apparent parallels in the conditions underpinning the recent revival of genetic theories and those giving rise to the earlier eugenicist ideas, then, one should not be distracted from recognising the distinctive rationalities of rule associated with the new genetics. Whereas within the older eugenics movement the focus was on populations and coercive control, with the new genetics the emphasis is on individuals and on counselling and individual choice (Conrad 1997). Genetic research and technologies are seen to obey the logic of the market, driven by the demand of 'consumers' for access to knowledge and technologies that will assist them in their efforts to maximise their health. This is not to say that the focus on populations has disappeared or that coercion has ceased. Rather, the emphasis on state responsibility and coercive ('top-down') intervention has been replaced by an emphasis on individual responsibility and self-care. In line with the imperatives of active citizenship, noted above, individuals are expected to play a role in monitoring and managing their own genetic risk. They are told that they must keep themselves informed about genes and how they affect one's health, as a new duty of the responsible citizen (Love 1996: 21). Being an informed decision maker entails 'weighing up' all available options: to undergo or forgo tests for known genetic 'defects' and, if found to have a 'defect', to undergo prescribed 'treatment' or simply to do nothing, to abort or not abort, and so on – and to consider attendant 'risks' and opportunities. In line with the imperatives of 'neo-liberal' rule, individuals are expected to manage their own relationship to risk, to adopt an actuarial or insurance-based approach to life. Actuarial or insurance-based reasoning, it has been noted by governmentality scholars, is increasingly apparent in a wide range of social institutions and contexts apart from public health and preventive medicine, including education, employment, crime control and personal and financial planning, emerging alongside and, in many cases, supplanting existing 'disciplinary technologies' of rule which employ coercive techniques for controlling errant individuals.

Pat O'Malley (1996) has drawn attention to the increasing privatisation of actuarialism – what he calls prudentialism – accompanying political interventions that seek to promote the increased play of market forces. For instance, in the area of health, as the field of publicly provided or subsidised health care is reduced and the range and scale of services provided by the state is narrowed, there has been a move to make qualifying conditions of access to services more rigorous, to promote private health insurance and provision of private medical services. At the same time, new regimes and routines of the body have come into play, 'founded on the assumption that subjects of risk will opt to participate in a self-imposed programme of health and fitness' (ibid.: 199). That is, *voluntary* participation in risk management has become an essential precondition of responsible selfhood:

> The rational individual will wish to become responsible for the self, for . . . this will produce the most palatable, pleasurable and effective mode of provision for security against risk. Equally, the responsible individual will take rational steps to avoid and to insure against risk, in order to be independent rather than a burden on others. Guided by actuarial data on risks (e.g. on smoking and lung cancer; bowel cancer and diet, etc.) and on the delivery of relevant services and expertise (e.g. relative costs and benefits of private and public medicine), the rational and responsible individual will take prudent risk-managing measures. Within such prudential strategies, then, calculative self-interest is articulated with acturialism to generate risk management as an everyday practice of the self.
>
> (O'Malley 1996: 199–200)

Genetic counselling

It is at this juncture that genetic counselling plays a key facilitative role. Genetic counselling adopts what has been called a 'non-directive' approach, which involves 'informing' people about risks, causes of illness and possible therapies so that they can arrive at their own decision (Beck-Gernsheim 1995: 92). The Danish Council of Ethics, for instance, suggests in a 1993 report that there is 'an obligation to help the weak which will be best exemplified when screening results in the curing of a serious disease' (see Chadwick and Levitt 1996). As Chadwick and Levitt (ibid.: 67) point out: 'in genetics, the duty to help has a special intention – to offer information that will facilitate autonomy'. According to the current rhetoric, people have a 'right to know' about their genetic risk, so that they can make an 'informed choice' about their health planning (see also Petersen 1998.) One health department pamphlet advises that a genetic counsellor can 'help you learn more about a hereditary condition' by:

- confirming or explaining a diagnosis;
- estimating the risk that you may have a child with the condition if it already occurs in your family;
- discussing with you the types of tests for the condition available before and/or during pregnancy;
- discussing ways of coping with the condition and the medical and social supports available; and
- identifying community resources that may be helpful.

It adds that 'a genetic counsellor can tell you how likely it is that a particular hereditary condition will recur if there is already a history in your family' (Hereditary Disease Unit 1995a). This approach is premised upon a model of rational decision making which assumes that, when properly advised about risk of genetic disease, individuals will weigh up all available information and arrive at the most appropriate decision. Genetic information, it is assumed, will make people more knowledgeable consumers, by allowing them to recognise their own vulnerability to genetic disease and to undertake appropriate preventive intervention.

To say that contemporary rationalities of rule emphasise agency is not equivalent to saying that subjects are unconstrained. As Steinberg (1997: 120) argues, the non-directive advice of experts is compromised (if not obviated) by the language of risks which permeates discourses of genetic screening and counselling. An emphasis on the costs for the community of genetic burden and the perceived economic and social benefits of modifying risks shape the context within which non-directive advice is offered and individual choice is exercised. Growing expectations surrounding the need for genetic testing are such that we may soon reach a situation where, if individuals know that certain genes cause disease and do not undergo testing where this is available, they are *irresponsible* for leaving things to chance (King 1995). The predictive information of risk assessment is seen to be of value to many contemporary institutions and organisations – schools, workplaces, the insurance industry, the health care industry, sports teams and the legal profession – who look for guidance in anticipating and controlling future contingencies. In societies increasingly preoccupied with cost containment and economic efficiency, it is seen as crucial that possible future eventualities are foreseen and opportunities exploited, or disbenefits anticipated and prevented. The popular appeal of genetics, indeed, lies in its image of being a predictive science – as providing a means to uncover predispositions (Nelkin and Lindee 1995: 165). In the United States at least, genetic testing is 'driven' by such groups as health insurers, who seek to avoid costly insurance payouts; physicians, who wish to protect themselves against malpractice suits; and employers, who aim to identify and exclude workers with specific traits that may predispose them to illness from exposure to certain chemical agents and thus avoid compensation claims and costly changes to the workplace environment (Nelkin 1992; Nelkin and Lindee 1995: 159–68).

One of the key promises of the Human Genome Project (HGP), launched in 1989 as a 10–15-year, US$3 billion effort to 'map' human genetic make-up, is to identify those genes that predispose us to disease and to uncover new treatment options for the individual. When the HGP began, it was claimed that there exist 5,000 or more human diseases that are genetically based. The effort to find the 'offending' genes and to develop appropriate therapies is seen by authorities as holding immense promise in illness prevention (Peters 1997). Genomics is also believed to have a benefit in the control of new strains of infectious diseases, which are expected to emerge as a result of the overuse of antibiotics. Geneticists are confident of deciphering the genomes of 50–100 micro-organisms, including the biggest killers such as TB, cholera and malaria (Venter and Cohen 1997). Prenatal tests are now available not just for life-threatening disorders but for conditions that are treatable after birth, for conditions that do not manifest until later in life, such as breast cancer, and other non-medical problems, such as homosexuality (Andrews 1996: 970). The new technology of fetal cell sorting is one of the new genetic technologies that is premised on the assumptions that women want the genetic information and that, since it is 'risk-free', it will readily find application in screening large populations of women (ibid.: 971). This technology is seen to provide fetal information without creating a *physical* risk to the fetus or the pregnant woman (which exists, say, with amniocentesis) and to offer more women the option of prenatal testing. It involves a 'simple' blood test on women and then laboratory analysis of minute quantities of fetal blood cells circulating in the woman's blood. Prenatal diagnosis is then undertaken on those cells to determine, for example, whether the fetus has Down's syndrome, cystic fibrosis, Tay-Sachs disease or other disorders. The growing availability of supposedly risk-free genetic technologies such as this, combined with the imperatives of responsible, 'healthy' citizenship, compromise the exercise of free choice in relation to genetic testing.

The discourse of the family responsibility

The ideal of non-directive advice in genetic counselling is also questioned by the existence of a pervasive discourse of family responsibility. Genetic counselling is premised on the assumption that subjects will be conscious of, and seek to fulfil, their responsibilities to present family members and future offspring. Increasingly, individuals are expected to inform themselves about the history of their family health, making use of reports from other family members and family friends, and of family records such as birth, marriage and death certificates. Many health departments are now advising people about the importance of knowing one's 'family health tree', and offering pamphlets which advise people how to find out whether or not there are any hereditary conditions in their family (see, e.g., Hereditary Disease Unit 1995b). This discourse bares a striking resemblance to the discourse of the family that characterised the older eugenics.

As Steinberg (1997: 75–6) notes, eugenics has been based upon assumptions of 'legitimate' kinship 'in which class, gendered and racialised inequalities are normalised and in which heterosexuality is assumed and (re)inscribed'. The operation of these assumptions was reflected, for instance, in Nazi responses to male homosexuals, who were seen as an immediate threat to the growth of the nation and were partly blamed for the lower birth rates, and hence subjected to various repressive measures (Grau 1995: 4). The family health tree used in public health today has an early antecedent in the family pedigree chart used in the US earlier this century to research the inheritance of a variety of physical, mental and personality traits, often based on highly subjective and impressionistic data collected from family members (Allen 1996: 24–5). Then, as now, prime responsibility for genetic health fell on women. With a falling birth rate and a high incidence of child mortality, women as bearers of children were in the front line of defence of the imperial race in many nation-states in western Europe. Motherhood was taught so that women would fulfil their primary, 'natural' purpose of replenishing and improving the human stock (Miles 1993: 69).

Within the new genetics, these compulsions are less apparent and less obviously punitive. Individuals are expected to be far more autonomous or 'self-directed'. However, the familial obligations assumed of the responsible subject, and the potential for the punishment of those who do not fulfil these obligations, are none the less evident, as underlined by a report of the Nuffield Council on Bioethics – 'UK's nearest equivalent to a national bioethics committee' – published in late 1993 (see Gillon 1994). While it affirms the need for the availability of 'non-directive' information, the Council also emphasises the individual's obligations to inform other family members about the results of the genetic screening that might be of major importance to them. Examples cited include the carrying of a gene for a severe disorder which alters their approach to reproduction (e.g. cystic fibrosis, thallassaemia or Tay-Sachs disease); or that may put them at risk of a genetic disorder whose manifestations may be fatal and preventable (e.g. familial colon cancer or breast cancer) or fatal and unpreventable (e.g. Huntington's disease). Where individuals are reluctant to pass on important genetic information to family members, the Council argues, it is the responsibility of health professionals to 'seek to persuade individuals, if persuasion should be necessary, to allow the disclosure of relevant genetic information to other family members'. Further, where such persuasion is considered unsuccessful, and where this 'may have serious implications for relatives', exceptionally 'the individual's desire for confidentiality may be over-ridden' (citing ibid.: 67).

Continuing faith in rational science

Despite the recent shift towards the rhetorics of active citizenship, rational science and rational management continue to play a crucial role in the resolution of problems in the new genetics. Within public health and the broader culture, genetic science is seen as generating objective data about the make-up of our corporeal bodies. Its object is the natural realm, which is viewed as separate from, and largely unaffected by, the cultural realm. The genetic research effort is underpinned by faith in the positivist premise that one can separate the knower from the known, or the subject from the object, and a view of science as a neutral activity, free of social and ethical values (Delanty 1997: 11–13). This premise has come under increasing question since the 1950s, creating what some have described as a 'crisis of epistemology', and this is reflected in concerns about the social purposes and consequences of genetic research. However, despite growing anxiety about the purposes and impacts of genetics, there has been relatively little systematic analysis of genetic research itself as a cultural production or as a political process. One of the contributions of poststructuralists has been to focus attention on the language and rationality of science, and to ask what particular images of bodies and selves are embedded in scientific theories and in descriptions about science, and what this reveals about the relations between power and knowledge. In scientists' accounts, genetic research is very often portrayed as a challenging and creative quest or 'hunt' to 'discover' 'faulty' or 'defective' genes, as is evident in the following description:

> To understand the enormous problem of finding a gene some-where on an individual's strand of DNA, imagine that a single human genome is long enough to circle the globe. On this scale, the amount of DNA in a chromosome would extend for a thousand miles. A gene would span just one twentieth of a mile, and a disease-causing defect – a point of mutation, a change in only one DNA base pair – could run as short as one twentieth of an inch. What we are thus searching for is comparable to a fraction of an inch on the circumference of the globe! In this immense morass of DNA, finding the exact address of a gene and pinpointing its fault makes for extremely tough going, and it requires all of the creativity and ingenuity of everyone engaged in the quest.
>
> (Wexler 1992: 212)

This description reveals a great deal about how culture shapes scientific accounts of nature. Deployment of the metaphor of the map (more specifically the global map) in this passage is common in the language of genetics, and reinforces the notion that science is a 'journey' involving 'discovery' or the revelation of some essential, underlying natural reality (i.e. 'finding the exact address of the gene'). The HGP itself is described as a gene 'mapping' project. It involves the drawing of three kinds of 'maps': linkage maps, based on studies of family genealogies, which 'show which genes are reinherited and roughly where they are on the chromosomes'; physical maps, which identify the gene's location on the DNA; and sequence maps, which identify the series of base pairs on the physical map (Rabinow 1992: 238–9). This gene mapping allows boundaries to be drawn between the normal and the abnormal, the 'healthy' genes and the 'defective' or 'faulty' genes. In the above portrayal, the search for genetic 'faults' presents as an arduous or painstaking endeavour – a massive intelligence operation – requiring 'creativity' and 'ingenuity', thus reflecting a vision of the scientist as a problem solver rather than as a producer of the object of enquiry. It is a vision which reinforces the view of the separation of the observer from the observed and from his or her observation statements, and buttresses the power of experts, who are seen as disinterested interpreters of the 'truth' of our biological make-up.

In many accounts of genetic research, scientists are depicted as altruistic, working diligently in pursuit of knowledge, whose application will necessarily advance the greater 'good' of 'the public'. Indeed, genetic researchers sometimes describe themselves as involved in a crusade to relieve human misery, as seen in this excerpt from Robert Cook-Deegan's book, *The Gene Wars*:

> A geneticist can work for years in a laboratory, never seeing an affected patient or commiserating with an afflicted family. The daily laboratory routine is relatively stable, if intense and demanding. Once the impact of a disease is directly experienced – the pain and devastation it causes for specific people – laboratory work acquires a new meaning. It demands greater urgency. The stakes go up; the room for excuses and tolerance of delay go dramatically down. Laboratory manipulations become less an exercise in abstract problem-solving and more a holy crusade against a common enemy. Disease becomes evil; eradicating it a primary need. Medical research differs

from other scientific fields in this respect. It is driven by this passion for life – the hunger to understand life in order to preserve it.

(Cook-Deegan 1994: 24–5)

The deployment of military metaphors ('the enemy') and reference to disease as 'evil', apparent here, have a long history in bio-medicine and have helped legitimate invasive interventions into bodies while bolstering the status and power of the experts. Genetic scientists are frequently seen to be aligned with 'good' against an 'evil' enemy which needs to be 'eradicated'. Appeals to the preservation of life, also seen here, provide powerful legitimation for research, particularly that research which seeks to fortify the body's natural 'defences' (see below). It is significant that the HGP has its origins in concerns about the effects of mutational damage to atomic bomb survivors and on the health of future generations. Cook-Deegan – 'a close observer of the genome project . . . [and] at times a minor participant' (from 1986 to 1988 he was part of the team that prepared a report on the genome project for the US Congress) – traces 'several roots' of the human genome project back to the Manhattan District Project to build an atomic bomb. As he explains, some of these roots led through studies to determine if there would be 'a final, genetic wave of effects' (inherited mutations) from exposure to the bombs at Hiroshima and Nagasaki. Others, he says, can be traced through the mathematicians who helped create the initial atomic bomb and then, after the Second World War, the hydrogen fusion bomb (Cook-Deegan 1994: 92–106).

Against the view of science as objective, as a process of discovery, as libratory and as altruistic, a growing number of writers have presented an alternative view of science as value-laden, as productive of its objects, as regulative, and as shaped by commercial interests and personal career aspirations. In particular, the idea that one can gain direct, unmediated access to knowledge, or what is known as the 'metaphysics of presence', has been critiqued across diverse fields of thought. The attempt to develop an objective 'view from nowhere' is seen to be not only unrealisable but as having exclusionary implications (see, e.g., Haraway 1991; Young 1990). Many feminists, historians, philosophers and sociologists of science have pointed out that natural knowledge and cultural knowledge are inseparable, and hence descriptions of 'nature' are bound to reflect broader visions of society, theories of causation and notions of individual and social responsibility. For instance, there has been a growing corpus of (mainly Foucauldian-inspired) research showing how the supposedly stable facts about the sexes as embodied dualities reflect cultural assumptions about gender (see, e.g., Butler 1993; Hausman 1995; Laqueur 1990). Work such as this shows that, rather than providing unmediated access to 'real', corporeal bodies, scientific knowledge and practices *fabricate* bodies. As one of the major languages of modern biology, genetic science has helped forge a radically new understanding of the body and of its functioning – an image which suggests that individual destinies are written into the genes which can be 'read' like a horoscope to reveal our ultimate fates. Genetic science is seen not only to reveal the workings of nature, but also to offer the possibility of controlling what nature has bequeathed 'us'. Thus endeavours to 'correct' 'faulty' genes in the body cells of living individuals ('somatic therapy') and to alter germ cells in the attempt to influence heredity and improve the quality of future generations ('germline therapy') reveal faith in the arbitrating powers of science (Peters 1997).

Remaking the body

For most of the last one hundred years or so, the biomedical view of the body has predominated. Within the biomedical framework, the body is likened to a machine with interrelated parts which are liable to breakdown that can be corrected through the application of rational science. The mechanical view of the body was developed during a period in which physics was beginning to provide the master metaphor for understanding the functioning of society as well as the processes of nature, and the workings of industrial society were seen to have their counterpart in the workings of the human body. It is a metaphor which has both legitimated the intervention into bodies of a certain group of experts (doctors) and has constructed the patient as largely blameless and passive, as a victim of circumstances beyond his or her control. Threats to bodily integrity (i.e. 'germs') are seen to lie just *outside* the body, in the external physical environment: in the home, workplace, clothing, surfaces of the body, and so on (Martin 1994: 24). Germ theory presupposes the existence of a central administrative machinery for monitoring disease outbreaks, surveilling the population and eradicating sources of infection. This view of the body has strongly shaped the conception and practices of public health through most of the nineteenth and twentieth centuries. The understanding of disease as infection that arose from and was strengthened in unhealthy locales and then transmitted through the air (i.e. miasmas) led in the nineteenth century to strategies that focus on regulating sites of disease and the means of its circulation (Rabinow 1989: 34–5). The contagion theory of nineteenth-century public health postulated that disease was transmitted by direct bodily contact, and so the prevention of contact of bodies was the basic defence. It was seen as the duty of government to intervene at this crucial point in the causation of disease through the implementation of various sanitary measures (Pelling 1993: 321–2). The *cordon sanitaire* was the classic means of separating bodies and spaces; however, this approach was increasingly supplanted in the early twentieth century by the application of new methods of 'hygiene' for safeguarding the defences of the body.

Although this nineteenth-century mechanical view of the body persists, the new genetics reflects and reinforces a view of the body as a cybernetic organism. This is a machine endowed with its own purpose: autonomous, capable of constructing itself, maintaining itself and reproducing itself (Keller 1992: 113). As Keller explains, the primary purpose of this machine is its own survival or, more accurately, the survival and reproduction of DNA that is said to both 'program' and direct its operation. In Dawkins's description, the organism is a 'survival machine' that has been constructed to house its genes, which have as their primary property inherent 'selfishness' (citing ibid.: 114). This conception of the body mirrors the view of the self as atomistic, entrepreneurial and self-responsible. The development of a notion of the body as an autonomous, self-sustaining system in the latter half of the twentieth century, and the corresponding decline of concerns about external threats to the integrity of the body ('keeping the germs away'), has been noted by Emily Martin (1994) in her study of the role of immunity in American culture. As Martin (ibid.: 33) notes:

> As the interior [of the body] comes into focus, concern with hygiene and the cleanliness of the outside surfaces of the body diminishes. It is as if, whatever is out there, and however deadly and dirty it is, the body's interior lines of defense will be able to handle it. By the time we reach accounts in contemporary biology and health books ... the interior of the body has

been enormously elaborated. 'Recognition' of disease-causing microbes is fantastically honed and refined and the immune system 'tailors' highly specific responses that can be almost unimaginably various. Drawing on an immense, genetically generated, and constantly changing arsenal of resources, the body can hardly rely on mere habit any longer.

Within many recent descriptions, the body is portrayed as 'naturally' well-equipped to ward off infection, to meet whatever challenges and threats it might encounter. As Martin notes, in both scientific and popular accounts, the body is portrayed as specialised but 'flexible' – reflecting an ideal currently shaping diverse areas of economic and social organisation; for example, the ability of labour markets and the process of labour to adapt to changing conditions of production (ibid.: 40). One of the goals of genetic research is to develop genetic therapies in order to make the body even more resiliant and adaptable. This can be achieved by introducing a gene to compensate for the 'faulty' gene responsible for the disease (Steinberg 1997: 113). Recent efforts to develop 'chemical keys' to 'switch off defective genes' that cause inherited diseases such as sickle-cell anaemia and cystic fibrosis reflect a vision of the perfectible body. The assumption is that if researchers are able to locate 'vulnerable sites and understand how harm is done, they can look for ways to protect DNA from damage' (Thomas 1998: 37).

The impact of genetics, however, extends far beyond its supposed health benefits. The lines between the applications of genetic knowledge for prevention or treatment of disease and non-health applications for enhancement or control of traits is becoming increasingly blurred. An example of the blurring of the lines between health and non-health applications of genetics can be seen clearly in the case of human growth hormone treatment. This treatment was originally developed for people with an inherited hormone deficiency, but is now also prescribed in some countries for short, healthy children to help them grow (Boyce 1997). Boyce notes that of the hundreds of gene therapy trials undertaken on thousands of patients since 1990, 'only a few dozen of them have involved diseases caused by defects in single genes'. Most researchers are working on multigene disorders, such as cancers, infectious diseases and non-fatal conditions such as arthritis and, since characteristics such as appearance and personality are also believed to be determined by more than one gene, there is some concern that multigene research will eventually lead to the genetic manipulation of these traits. It has been suggested that companies will seek approval for enhancement gene therapies by disguising them as medical therapies. For example, a therapy to improve memory might claim only to prevent Alzheimers. As Boyce (ibid.: 20) argues, the ultimate impact of gene therapies on future generations has yet to be determined, but it could well be that inserted genes may find their way into sperm or eggs and affect future generations.

The new genetic conception of the body reflects an essentialist understanding of human identity. That is, health problems and social behaviours are seen to be an intrinsic aspect of the person, with any faults ultimately being located in the individual. Although many, if not most, geneticists acknowledge some causative role for the environment in genetic health, genetics-based public health shifts the focus away from the environmental determinants that have been central to public health discourse and locates the 'cause' of disease squarely with the individual. As Steinberg (1997: 117) argues in her recent analysis of genetic language, notions of inherent abnormality and blame are integral to many contemporary descriptions of genetic disease. The use of terms such as 'genetic defect' and 'genetic disorder' identify the problem as intrinsic to the very body of the person affected: 'genetic disease is not only something terrible that someone *has*, but something someone *is*' (emphases in original):

> More emphatically than the theory of germs as cause of disease, with genes the 'foreign agent' of disease is incorporated in and of, indeed intrinsic to the very body of the person affected. In this context an 'offending gene' implicitly bespeaks an 'offensive' person, and is clearly implicated in the putatively imperative logic of genetic screening as a strategy to prevent the birth of persons with such 'diseases'.

> (Ibid.)

The concept of DNA as a boundary marker and a source of true identity has found a practical application in the development of 'genetic fingerprinting'. As Nelkin and Lindee (1995: 46–7) explain, the public and judicial enthusiasm for this means of identification attests to the significance of DNA as an icon, or metaphor, for describing the essence of a person, and popular descriptions emphasise the awesome power of this scientific technique for sorting and identification. Genetic fingerprinting was originally developed in the early 1980s as a 'foolproof' means of identifying criminals by studying DNA in biological materials found at the crime scene and comparing it with the DNA of the suspect for the presence of specific DNA sequences known to vary in human populations. Since 1987, when it was used to help solve a widely publicised British murder case, it has become a powerful form of evidence in court, and has been heralded in the press as the 'single greatest forensic breakthrough since the advent of fingerprinting at the turn of the century'. Although DNA fingerprinting is not infallible, in popular stories it is portrayed as the 'ultimate identifier', as providing uncontentious proof of the essence and identity of the person (ibid.: 47). Thus, the current media image of the genetic fingerprint is 'the barcode that can be read at the checkout' (Strathern 1995: 103).

Governing one's own genetic fate

In the expert literature, there has been substantial discussion about how best to persuade those who are deemed to be most genetically at risk to recognise their own genetic risk and to act responsibly on that information. That is, the problem is conceived as one of how to make subjects more effective governors of their own genetic fates. One of the chief problems that has been identified is lay people's ignorance of science and of the mathematics of chance or probability (Kerr *et al.* 1998a). In genetics, as in other areas of science, scientists and other commentators see ignorance as a deficit that needs to be corrected through more or better information. There has been little apparent recognition of the fact that public ignorance is actively constructed and few efforts to understand what lay people's apparent ignorance might reveal about their relationship to science (Michael 1996). People's ignorance of the 'correct facts' is frequently seen as a problem of people's interpretative processes and/or of the way information is conveyed, apparent in the comments of a clinical psychologist, who has studied and worked with sufferers of Huntington's disease in Venezuela:

> I am always surprised by the imaginative ways in which people can misinterpret genetic information. One common and very understandable mistake is the belief that at least one person in every family [with Huntington's disease] will be sick. In the Huntington's disease testing programs [undertaken in

Venezuela], people often arrive with the conviction that whether they will or will not get the disease depends on the fate of siblings. If my siblings are sick, my risk goes down; if they are old and healthy, my risk goes up. This is a perfectly reasonable misinterpretation given the way in which genetic inheritance is usually explained. Most genetic textbooks and consumer pamphlets teach principles of inheritance by showing a family of four children and two parents in which two children are affected and two are not. And doctors often explain risks by saying 'half your children' or 'one-quarter of your children will become sick'. You must always say, 'Each child has a fifty-fifty or 25 percent risk, regardless of the rest of the family.'

(Wexler 1992: 234–5)

The remedy suggested here, improved communication, is a commonly recommended panacea for problems of 'misinterpretation' in genetic counselling, and effectively casts aside any doubt about the validity or value of genetic information. There is no acknowledgement of the difficulties and uncertainties surrounding the interpretation of genetic data, or disagreements about the significance of test results, or that 'except for a few diagnostic genetic tests, most fall into a gray area where the results can be more confusing than helpful' (Feldman 1996: 15; see also Malinowski 1994: 1512–13). In most cases, it is simply assumed that the supposedly objective knowledge of science is superior to the subjective or interpretative knowledge of lay people, and that if people are to make properly 'informed choices' they need to be educated or advised about the 'correct' scientific 'facts'.

In genetic counselling, there is little recognition of lay people's own 'stock of knowledge' about the new genetics, which is derived from the media and other sources and from their own direct personal experiences of genetic illness. In one study, drawing on data from ten focus groups carried out in central Scotland in 1996, it was found that lay people draw on diverse sources of knowledge about science and genetics in making sense of the new genetics, and that their accounts are broadly related to their health (including their hereditary status), their class, age and gender (Kerr *et al.* 1998a). While people did not always have a full and detailed understanding of the technical processes involved, many did have a basic technical knowledge of genetics, generally linked to notions of heredity of physical characteristics and disease. They were also likely to have a general awareness of methodological issues, particularly around the fallibility of testing, the iatrogenic effects of prenatal testing (e.g. the risk of miscarriage associated with amniocentesis), and the difficulties associated with scientific proof, as well as knowledge of the institutional aspects of science and medicine that pertain to the new genetics, such as issues to do with the politics of funding, the relations between scientists, and the relationship between the new genetics, pharmaceutical companies and government. But, as would be expected, the breadth and depth of understanding that people have, and can draw on when discussing the new genetics, were found to be closely related to their social location. For example, women have more experiences of prenatal testing than men, and this featured in their accounts of their views about genetic testing; and people with disabilities shared unpleasant memories of being disregarded or devalued by the medical professionals, which were reflected in their views on eugenics (ibid.: 51). As the researchers concluded, calls for an 'informed public' to participate in debates about the new genetics, which one finds frequently in policy discussions, are based on questionable assumptions about public ignorance and people's inability or unwillingness to participate (ibid.: 57).

Contesting the imperatives of genetic health

If one is serious about questioning these assumptions, I believe one must pay greater attention to lay people's own everyday knowledge and rationalities. Lay knowledges could provide the basis for exploring the contradictions and tensions around genetic knowledge and genetic treatment and prevention and for contesting the imperatives surrounding genetic health. By attending to the rationalities employed by lay people in decision making in relation to the new genetics and to the impact of social contexts within which their accounts are articulated, the new genetics could become an important site for contesting the meanings of citizenship. If there is to be a shift away from the 'deficit' model of public understanding of science in general and genetics in particular, it is essential to explore how lay people engage with, analyse and utilise knowledge. Recognition needs to be given to the complexities of lay accounts of genetic science, including acknowledgement of the uncertainties often ignored in expert accounts. As Kerr *et al.* (1998b) argue, when professionals make appeals to individual choice they often contrast their present-day practices, which constitute the 'gold standard', with those of the past or the future, where constraints, such as access to genetic information, might limit clients' autonomy. In making such claims they are suggesting that current practices support individual choice for clients, and are focusing attention away from the clinic to the wider society. Lay people's accounts are more diverse than those of professionals because they neither share the professionals' resources nor their interests in protective boundary maintenance (ibid.: 131). In their own study of lay accounts of the new genetics, Kerr *et al.* (ibid.) outlined some of the complexities involved in the 'drawing of the line' between acceptable and unacceptable research and practice in the new genetics which tend to be obscured in expert accounts. As they note, such accounts could be an important resource for critical discussion about the new genetics and for raising questions which tend to be ignored in policy discussions.

Such a strategy would entail giving credence to lay people's differing accounts of genetic risk and what these accounts might reveal about the public's relationship to science in general and genetics in particular. The frequent claim that lay people are ignorant about their genetic risk, noted above – generally expressed in counselling as a gambling odd – rests on the dubious premise that people are poor at grasping odds or probabilities. This denies subjects' practical knowledge of probability derived from the rich tradition of betting found among a broad segment of the population (Macintyre 1995). As Macintyre points out, the calculation of odds are a routine part of betting in games of chance, horses, dogs, football and in investment decisions such as 'playing' the stock market and planning and saving for one's future financial security. Participation in such games and planning involves often complex calculations of probabilities and decisions in cost-benefit ratios ('what stake to put on what odds') (ibid.: 229). Prudentialism, or the privatisation of risk management, mentioned earlier, indeed implies that the responsible subject will be reasonably familiar with the mathematics of chance. This is likely to constitute part of 'lay epidemiology', or assessment of health risk (Davison *et al.* 1991), based on everyday observations of cases of illness and death in personal networks and the public arena, which may involve the fatalist conclusion that it is best simply to 'leave things to chance'. Indeed, the strong determinist image of genetics – the view that our fates are written into our genes – suggests that a rational response to genetic information might be to disregard what the experts say and do nothing. In other words, 'bad' genes is just 'bad luck'.

Serious attention to lay knowledges would involve recognising the complexities and ambiguities surrounding decision making in relation to genetic information, and the ways in which 'choices' are shaped by culture, gender, age, religion and social context. What empirical evidence exists suggests that there is likely to be a significant mismatch between expected rational practices of the self and subjects' participation in preventative behaviours. For instance, in relation to Huntington's disease it has been found that, at least in some genetic services, only a small proportion of people from families with a history of the disease take up the option of genetic testing, which is considered by the experts to be the most rational path for those deemed to be at risk (Macintyre 1995). In public health, it has been assumed that people might want to know their diagnosis so that they can avoid passing the condition on to their offspring, and so that they can plan their lives. However, many people have sought testing later in life when they could be expected to develop the disease and when it is too late to make decisions on child bearing or on career planning. Furthermore, some of those who have been found *not* to have the condition have experienced psychological distress and social disruption, in addition to relief in hearing the diagnosis. Other research has revealed that some women who have been informed that they are unlikely to have the gene for breast or ovarian cancer have found it difficult to believe this, and have wanted to continue with routine surveillance and, in some cases, plan for prophylactic surgery such as mastectomy (ibid.: 226–7). For pregnant women who are known carriers of 'bad' genes, the only available treatment or preventive option at present is to have an abortion. In a strong pronatalist context or where beliefs about the sanctity of life override any notion of a woman's right to abortion, termination of a pregnancy may not be considered to be an option. In such cases, medical knowledge of genetic disease either may not be sought at all or, when offered, may be contested or ignored.

The importance of paying heed to cultural values and social context is emphasised by research undertaken by Shirley Hill, which focused on the reproductive decision making of low-income African American mothers of children with sickle-cell disease (SCD), a group of blood disorders described in genetic screening programmes as 'serious and incurable, often causing early death' (Hill 1994: 30).

As Hill explains, education and screening programmes have been premised on a health belief model which assumes that persons diagnosed as having the sickle cell trait will alter their reproductive behaviours. However, this model fails to acknowledge the sociocultural context shaping health decisions. Although advocates of SCD programmes recognise and try to address the racism that underlies inadequate medical responses to SCD, they attempt to solve the problem by embracing free and voluntary screening to solve the problem, thereby effectively ignoring the influence of class and gender inequalities on women's responses to screening programmes (ibid.: 30–1). The options presented by screening programmes – screening both mothers and fathers, and forgoing parenthood – are not feasible for the low-income African American women as they do not have enough power in their relationships with men to insist that they be screened for SCD, or have access to adequate health care or prochoice attitudes towards abortion. In Hill's view, motherhood is seen as one of the few 'status-attaining and satisfying options' available, and the women are unwilling to sacrifice their right to have children for the sake of the SCD campaign. SCD medical knowledge is seen by the women to pose a threat to their reproductive autonomy and as a mandate, however subtle, to alter their reproductive behaviour. The health belief model did not coincide with the realities of life for these women, and they responded by obfuscating medical knowledge. As Hill concludes, 'in their view, medical knowledge did not represent the definitive truth and, by their health standards, SCD was not quite as dreadful as medical science suggested' (ibid.: 43–4). This study highlights the inadequacy of simple models of social behaviour and the complexities and tensions surrounding social action that are too often ignored by policy makers.

Rethinking 'policy'

Developments in the new genetics, outlined in this chapter, underline the limits of simple, reactive conceptions of policy, and the need for policy makers to develop more sophisticated approaches based upon recognition of the generative power of policy. The knowledges and practices of the new genetics are rapidly altering views of the body and the self, and giving rise to new kinds of problems to be managed and new forms of regulation and intervention; for example, requests for genetic information, screening of

populations, the creation of new genetic data banks, the education of the genetically 'at risk', the application of new therapies to
those with 'faulty' genes, and so on. These developments are under-
mining established notions of the natural and the normal, and hence
of 'health' and 'disease', while at the same time serving to bring
into question the subject/object, mind/body and fact/value dualisms
underlying the positivist scientific method. The supposed objectivity
of the 'facts' generated by genetic science is challenged by mounting
evidence showing just how profoundly the concept of nature is
shaped by culture. The language of the new genetics, articulated
above in the accounts of researchers and counsellors, reveals how
cultural values and ideals pervade thinking and practices and reinforce particular kinds of relations between experts and non-experts.
Embedded within the discourses and practices of the new genetics
are assumptions about how individuals should conduct themselves,
about their rationality, about their awareness of their bodies, about
how they should relate to experts, and about their responsibilities to others, including members of their immediate family and
future offspring. The new genetics would seem to illustrate clearly
the recent broadening of the concept of citizenship noted within
many contemporary societies, involving an emphasis on 'duties
implied by rights', which extend beyond one's own generation
(see Roche 1992).

To focus on the productive power of public health, it should be
emphasised, is not to deny the materiality of those conditions that
have traditionally been the focus of public health policies, nor is it
to suggest that public health policies and practices do not have
substantial impacts on individual bodies and lives. Quite the
contrary. Recent developments in genetic-based public health underline the power of knowledge to profoundly shape how human beings
construct and respond to their physical and social environments,
how they experience their own and others' bodies, and what they
perceive as the possibilities for social action and social change. With
the increasing 'geneticisation' of society it has become increasingly
difficult for people to ignore genetic information, because it has
become ubiquitous (particularly in the mainstream media and in
popular culture), and is likely to become increasingly so under the
influence of the HGP and other similar projects. People are forced
to confront and consider the implications of the claim that what
happens *inside* their bodies as a consequence of their biological
make-up is at least as important as, if not more important than, what

happens *to* their bodies as a result of external, physical and social environments. Indeed, as I have argued, the responsible citizen is *obliged* to reflect upon his or her own genetic health, to weigh up known risks and opportunities, and to choose among prescribed options, which may involve, apart from testing and counselling, submitting to intrusive and constant surveillance; changing life-style, including patterns of work and leisure; and undergoing 'treatment', including surgery (e.g. prophylactic mastectomy) or having an abortion. The new genetics has inaugurated at least a partial reconfiguring of public health as a domain of knowledge and practice, with less emphasis than in the past on 'health' as a product of the interactions between subjects and determining physical and social environments, and on forms of collective action focusing on *social* reform, and greater emphasis on perfecting bodies and on self-subjection.

The dominance of the reactive conception of policy has led policy analysts to overlook the impact on subjects and subjectivities of particular constructions of 'health', 'the public' and 'policy'. In discourses of public health, claims about the need to protect 'the public' from contagion have been, and continue to be, crucial in mobilising the support of populations for social regulations of one kind or other. Calls for such regulations tend to be based upon essentialist concepts of society and self, and involve the drawing of dualistic distinctions between groups: the pure/the impure, the innocent/the guilty, the careful/the careless, the risk avoider/ the risk taker, the responsible/the irresponsible, etc. Thus, those who are seen as having a genetic 'fault' or 'defect' and who do not conduct themselves according to the norms of 'healthy', responsible citizenship are likely to be labelled as irresponsible and as posing a danger to others and, as such, subject to new, insidious forms of regulation, including the demand that they submit themselves to 'treatment', including abortion. Responses to genetic illness illustrate how policies and practices 'designed' to prevent illness can give rise to fear, intolerance of the 'other' and social inequality. As Markel (1992: 214) notes, like quarantines in the past, new disease labels generated by the HGP not only provide barriers for protection against disease, but also create images of impaired function, aberrancy and diminished self-image. As scientific enquiry progresses and programmes such as the HGP generate new information, the potential for discrimination against and ostracism of those with 'undesirable' traits is likely to increase. The reductionism that is associated with the privileging of genetic knowledge diverts attention from the social, ethical and legal impacts of public health interventions. Recent developments in genetics underline the need for policy makers to rethink theoretical approaches to policy. In particular, there is a need for a thoroughgoing analysis of the rationalities implicit in policies and of implications for conceptions of self and citizenship. In this endeavour, poststructuralism offers useful tools of analysis and raises questions that have hitherto been largely neglected in both 'mainstream' and critical public health literature.

References

Allen, G. (1996) 'Science misapplied: the eugenic age revisited', *Technology Review*, August/September: 23–31.

Andrews, L.B. (1996) 'Prenatal screening and the culture of motherhood', *Hastings Law Journal*, 47, 4: 967–1006.

Ashton, J. and Seymour, H. (1988) *The New Public Health: The Liverpool Experience*, Milton Keynes: Open University Press.

Badinter, E. (1995) *XY: On Masculine Identity*, New York: Columbia University Press.

Bauman, Z. (1997) *Postmodernity and its Discontents*, Cambridge: Polity Press.

Beck-Gernsheim, E. (1995) *The Social Implications of Bioengineering*, Atlantic Highlands, NJ: Humanities Press.

Bogard, W. (1996) *The Simulation of Surveillance: Hypercontrol in Telematic Societies*, Cambridge: Cambridge University Press.

Boyce, N. (1997) 'In sickness and in death', *New Scientist*, 25 October, no. 2105: 20–1.

Bracht, N. (1991) 'Citizen participation in community health: principles for effective partnerships', in B. Badura and I. Kickbusch (eds), *Health Promotion Research: Towards a New Social Epidemiology*, WHO Regional Publications, European Series no. 37, London: WHO.

Bracht, N. and Tsouros, A. (1990) 'Principles and strategies of effective community participation', *Health Promotion International*, 5, 3: 199–208.

Bunton, R. (1998) 'Inequalities in late-modern health care', in A. Petersen and C. Waddell (eds), *Health Matters: A Sociology of Illness, Prevention and Care*, Sydney: Allen and Unwin; Sydney and Buckingham: Open University Press.

Butler, J. (1993) *Bodies That Matter: On the Discursive Limit of 'Sex'*, New York: Routledge.

Chadwick, R. and Levitt, M. (1996) 'Euroscreen: ethical and philosophical issues of genetic screening in Europe', *Journal of the Royal College of Physicians of London*, 30, 1: 67–9.

Christen, Y. (1991) *Sex Differences: Modern Biology and the Unisex Fallacy*, New Brunswick, NJ: Transaction Publishers.

Conrad, P. (1997) 'Public eyes and private genes: historical frames, news constructions, and social problems', *Social Problems*, 44, 2: 139–54.

Cook-Deegan, R. (1994) *The Gene Wars: Science, Politics, and the Human Genome*, New York: W.W. Norton.

Crossley, M.A. (1996) 'Choice, conscience, and context', *Hastings Law Journal*, 47, 4: 1223–39.

Daniel, C. (1996) 'Every baby a perfect baby?' *New Statesman*, 2 August: 20–2.

Davison, C., Davey Smith, G. and Frankel, S. (1991) 'Lay epidemiology and the prevention paradox: the implications of coronary candidacy for health education', *Sociology of Health and Illness*, 13, 1: 1–19.

Dawkins, R. (1976) *The Selfish Gene*, Oxford: Oxford University Press.

Delanty, G. (1997) *Social Science: Beyond Constructivism and Realism*, Buckingham: Open University Press.

Dikötter, F. (1998) *Imperfect Conceptions: Medical Knowledge, Birth Defects and Eugenics in China*, London: Hurst & Co.

Draper, E. (1993) 'Privacy rights, stigma, and genetic screening', *Forum for Applied Research and Public Policy*, Fall: 19–22.

Feldman, M.K. (1996) 'Genetic screening: not just another blood test', *Minnesota Medicine*, 79 (October): 14–17.

Flinn, M.W. (1965) *The Sanitary Condition of the Labouring Population of Great Britain, by Edwin Chadwick*, Edinburgh: Edinburgh University Press.

Foucault, M. (1991) 'Governmentality', in G. Burchell, C. Gordon and P. Miller (eds), *The Foucault Effect: Studies in Governmentality*, London: Harvester Wheatsheaf.

Frenk, J. (1993) 'The new public health', *Annual Review of Public Health*, 14: 469–90.

Garland, D. (1997) ' "Governmentality" and the problem of crime: Foucault, criminology, sociology', *Theoretical Criminology*, 1, 2: 173–214.

Gaulding, J. (1995) 'Race, sex, and genetic discrimination in insurance: what's fair?' *Cornell Law Review*, 80, 6: 1646–94.

Gillon, R. (1994) 'Ethics of genetic screening: the first report of the Nuffield Council on Bioethics', *Journal of Medical Ethics*, 20: 67–8.

Grau, G. (1995) *Hidden Holocaust? Gay and Lesbian Persecution in Germany 1933–45*, London: Cassell.

Hacking, I. (1986) 'Making up people', in T.C. Heller, M. Sosna and D.E. Wellberg (eds), *Reconstructing Individualism: Autonomy, Individuality, and the Self in Western Thought*, Stanford, CA: Stanford University Press.

Hacking, I. (1990) *The Taming of Chance*, Cambridge: Cambridge University Press.

Hamer, D. and Copeland, P. (1994) *The Science of Desire: The Search for the Gay Gene and the Biology of Behaviour*, New York: Simon and Schuster.

Haraway, D.J. (1991) *Simians, Cyborgs, and Women: The Reinvention of Nature*, New York: Routledge.

Hausman, B. (1995) *Changing Sex: Transsexualism, Technology, and the Idea of Gender*, Durham, NC: Duke University Press.

Hereditary Disease Unit (1995a) *Your Genetic Counselling Appointment*, pamphlet produced by Hereditary Disease Unit, Disease Control, Health Department of Western Australia, with assistance from Genetic Counselling Services, Birth Defects Registry and Health Promotion Services, Perth.

Hereditary Disease Unit (1995b) *Check Your Family Health Tree*, pamphlet produced by the Hereditary Disease Unit, Disease Control, Health Department of Western Australia.

Hill, S.A. (1994) 'Motherhood and the obfuscation of medical knowledge: the case of sickle cell disease', *Gender and Society*, 8, 1: 29–47.

Keller, E. Fox (1992) *Secrets of Life, Secrets of Death: Essays on Language, Gender and Science*, New York: Routledge.

Kerr, A., Cunningham-Burley, S. and Amos, A. (1998a) 'The new genetics and health: mobilizing lay expertise', *Public Understanding of Science*, 7, 1: 41–60.

Kerr, A., Cunningham-Burley, S. and Amos, A. (1998b) 'Drawing the line: an analysis of lay people's discussions about the new genetics', *Public Understanding of Science*, 7, 2: 113–33.

Kevles, D.J. (1995) *In the Name of Eugenics: Genetics and the Uses of Human Heredity*, Cambridge, MA: Harvard University Press.

King, D. (1995) 'The state of eugenics', *New Statesman and Society*, 25 August: 25–6.

Kohn, M. (1995) *The Race Gallery: The Return of Racial Science*, London: Jonathan Cape.

Laqueur, T. (1990) *Making Sex: Body and Gender from the Greeks to Freud*, Cambridge, MA: Harvard University Press.

Lewin, R. (1993) 'Genes from a disappearing world', *New Scientist*, 29 May: 25–9.

Love, R. (1996) 'Knowing your genes', *Public Understanding of Science*, 5, 1: 21–7.

Macintyre, S. (1995) 'The public understanding of science or the scientific understanding of the public? A review of the social context of the "new genetics"', *Public Understanding of Science*, 4, 3: 223–32.

Malinowski, M.J. (1994) 'Coming into being: law, ethics, and the practice of prenatal genetic screening', *Hastings Law Journal*, 45, 6: 1435–1526.

Markel, H. (1992) 'The stigma of disease: implications of genetic screening', *American Journal of Medicine*, 93: 209–15.

Martin, E. (1994) *Flexible Bodies: Tracking Immunity in American Culture – From the Days of Polio to the age of AIDS*, Boston, MA: Beacon Press.

Michael, M. (1996) 'Ignoring science: discourses of ignorance in the public understanding of science', in A. Irwin and B. Wynne (eds), *Misunderstanding Science? The Public Reconstruction of Science and Technology*, Cambridge: Cambridge University Press.

Miles, R. (1993) *Racism After 'Race Relations'*, London: Routledge.

Nelkin, D. (1992) 'The social power of genetic information', in D.J. Kevles and L. Hood (eds), *The Code of Codes: Scientific and Social Issues in the Human Genome Project*, Cambridge, MA: Harvard University Press.

Nelkin, D. and Lindee, M.S. (1995) *The DNA Mystique: The Gene as a Cultural Icon*, New York: W.H. Freeman.

Nørgaard-Pedersen, B. (1994) 'Towards acceptable practices for antenatal and neonatal screening for disease or disease risk', *Clinical Genetics*, 46: 152–9.

O'Malley, P. (1996) 'Risk and responsibility', in A. Barry, T. Osborne and N. Rose (eds), *Foucault and Political Reason: Liberalism, Neo-liberalism and Rationalities of Government*, London: UCL Press.

Osborne, T. (1997) 'Of health and statecraft', in A. Petersen and R. Bunton (eds), *Foucault, Health and Medicine*, London: Routledge.

Pasquino, P. (1991) 'Theatrum politicum: the genealogy of capital – police and the state of prosperity', in G. Burchell, C. Gordon and P. Miller (eds), *The Foucault Effect: Studies in Governmentality*, London: Harvester Wheatsheaf.

Pelling, M. (1993) 'Contagion/germ theory/specificity', in W.F. Bynam and R. Porter (eds), *Companion Encyclopedia of the History of Medicine*, vol. 1, London: Routledge.

Peters, T. (1997) *Playing God? Genetic Determinism and Human Freedom*, New York: Routledge.

Petersen, A. (1996) 'The "healthy" city, expertise, and the regulation of space', *Health and Place*, 2, 3: 157–65.

Petersen, A. (1998) 'The new genetics and the politics of public health', *Critical Public Health*, 8, 1: 79–91.

Petersen, A. and Lupton, D. (1996) *The New Public Health: Health and Self in the Age of Risk*, Sydney: Allen and Unwin; and London: Sage.

Pike, D., O'Keefe, E. and Pike, S. (1990) 'Camden in the WHO Healthy Cities project', *The Planner*, no. 21 (September): 17–20.

Porter, R. (1993) 'Diseases of civilization', in W.F. Bynum and R. Porter (eds), *Companion Encyclopedia of the History of Medicine*, London: Routledge.

Rabinow, P. (1989) *French Modern: Norms and Forms of the Social Environment*, Cambridge, MA: MIT Press.

Rabinow, P. (1992) 'Artificiality and enlightenment: from sociobiology to biosociality', in J. Crary and S. Kwinter (eds), *Incorporations*, Zone 6, New York: Urzone.

Rakiewicz, M. (1992) 'Remapping the human race', *Canadian Business*, August: 95–8.

Roche, M. (1992) *Rethinking Citizenship: Welfare, Ideology and Change in Modern Society*, Cambridge: Polity Press.

Rose, N. (1994) 'Regulating "the social"', in M. Valverde (ed.), *Radically Rethinking Regulation*, University of Toronto: Centre of Criminology, Toronto.

Rose, N. (1996) 'Governing "advanced" liberal democracies', in A. Barry, T. Osborne and N. Rose (eds), *Foucault and Political Reason: Liberalism, Neo-liberalism and Rationalities of Government*, London: UCL Press.

Rose, N. and Miller, P. (1992) 'Political power beyond the state: problematics of government', *British Journal of Sociology*, 43, 2: 173–205.

Rosen, G. (1974) *From Medical Police to Social Medicine: Essays on the History of Health Care*, New York: Science History Publications.

Steinberg, D.L. (1997) *Bodies in Glass: Genetics, Eugenics, Embryo Ethics*, Manchester: Manchester University Press.

Strathern, M. (1995) 'Nostalgia and the new genetics', in D. Battaglia (ed.), *Rhetorics of Self-making*, Berkeley, CA: University of California Press.

Thomas, J. (1998) 'Damage control', *New Scientist*, 7 February, no. 2120: 36–9.

Venter, C. and Cohen, D. (1997) 'Genetic code-breakers', *Weekend Australian*, 19–20 July: 28.

Wallerstein, N. (1993) 'Empowerment and health: the theory and practice of community change', *Community Development Journal*, 28, 3: 218–27.

Wexler, N. (1992) 'Clairvoyance and caution: repercussions from the Human Genome Project', in D.J. Kevles and L. Hood (eds), *The Code of Codes: Scientific and Social Issues in the Human Genome Project*, Cambridge, MA: Harvard University Press.

Wyld, D.C., Cappel, S.D. and Hallock, D.E. (1992) 'The new eugenics? Employers and genetic screening in the "risk society"', *Futures Research Quarterly*, Fall: 23–35.

Yeo, M. (1993) 'Toward an ethic of empowerment for health promotion', *Health Promotion International*, 8, 3: 225–35.

Young, I.M. (1990) *Justice and the Politics of Difference*, Princeton, NJ: Princeton University Press.

Question from Patricia: Alan, I think that the suggestions you make regarding lay knowledges are very important. But it strikes me that lay knowledges about genetics 'outside' scientific knowledge are impossible, given that genetics is a scientific project built on very specific expert technologies. So maybe it's a very different kind of lay knowledge you are talking about, something which offers an alternative way to thinking about health, risk, mortality, etc. Can you comment?

Response: Patricia, in the chapter I was trying to make the point that expert knowledges and practices are based on a rationality that tends to exclude lay knowledges, which I take to include the rationalities that people routinely employ in deciding among various courses of action. These rationalities may be quite complex and, from the professionals' point of view, may seem ambiguous and contradictory, indeed *irrational*. Professionals privilege scientific knowledge over other kinds of knowledge and employ a model of decision making that is abstract, in that it does not take account of how people actually make decisions in different situations or acknowledge the multiple constraints on decision making. This can be seen with health belief models which assume that, given the 'correct' information, people will alter their behaviour in a given direction. The options and possible lines of action, however, are preordained. The underlying premise is that experts know what is in people's best interests, and that decisions are unaffected by sociocultural contexts. The limitations of this model are underlined by the study I cited, involving African American mothers of children with sickle-cell disease: screening programmes were found to present options (screening both mothers and fathers, and forgoing parenthood) which were simply not viable in this particular situation, given the importance of motherhood and the power relations that exist between men and women. In genetic counselling, there is little apparent recognition of how sociocultural contexts shape perceptions of genetic risk and what are seen as the possibilities for action.

Lay knowledges about genetics incorporate scientific knowledge, but are by no means coextensive with scientific knowledge. Thus, there exists lay understandings about heredity and the hereditability of disease which is derived in part from science, at least as it is portrayed by the media and other sources, but also from the family (perhaps passed down through the generations), religion and other sources. To be sure, scientific knowledge infiltrates all levels of society. In our scientific and mass-mediated culture, it is impossible to insulate oneself from new scientific ideas. However, people's 'stock of knowledge' about genetics draws on a far more diverse range of sources than science, including personal observations about illness, risk and mortality. In some cases, this knowledge may conflict with scientific knowledge. As I have mentioned, lay conceptions of risk derived from experiences of gambling and from other sources may not concur with expert definitions of risk, which are usually expressed in genetic counselling as gambling odds. This is seen as a problem by counsellors, who tend to work with 'deficit' models of lay knowledge. If one is serious about recovering 'subjugated' or 'disqualified' knowledges from the hegemony of positivistic science – which I take to be one of the important potential contributions of poststructuralism – then one should challenge the tendency to dismiss the non-scientific accounts of lay people as indicators of ignorance. I have suggested that lay knowledges could provide the focus for an exploration of the contradictions around genetic knowledge and treatment and prevention, and for contesting the imperatives of genetic health. The very fact that little attention has thus far been given to these lay knowledges attests to the hegemony of scientific and professional knowledge in modern western society.

Question from Ian: Your essay argues that the new genetics is an important site at which the 'rationality of rule' of advanced liberalism is developed/applied, inasmuch as it inculcates a 'responsibility' to care for one's body/genome. You contrast this with lay people's everyday knowledges and rationalities – knowledges which could provide the basis for exploring the contradictions, etc. Could the recognition and development of such alternative knowledges be articulated in terms of a discourse and practice of citizenship alternative to that of advanced liberalism; and, if so, how might that be reflected in public health policy with respect to the development of the new genetics, both in relation to research programmes of the new genetics and the form of its application to clinical situations?

Response: A truly democratic polity, I believe, would allow for the generation and expression of a diverse range of lay knowledges. Lay knowledges of healing and of all kinds of problem solving would flourish, without undue interference and restriction by the 'experts' and political authorities. As it stands, only certain authorised rationalities and knowledges are permitted free play, and this denies the richness of how people actually conduct their lives and 'make do' within the systems that dominate them. Increasingly, citizenship is being cast in terms of *individual* rights and duties. With the 'winding back' of the welfare state in many contemporary societies, established rights of a *collective* nature have disappeared or are rapidly disappearing; for example, the right of collective bargaining and the right to work and to receive the 'safety net' of social security. Many minority group rights and women's rights have been substantially under-mined. In light of this, there is a need to rethink the meanings of citizenship, and to question the utility of this concept in efforts to protect or extend rights. I'm not sure whether it is feasible to articulate lay know-ledges in terms of a discourse and practice of citizenship that is *alternative* to that of neo-liberalism. My point is that the meanings of citizenship need to be opened to thorough scrutiny and that the non-expert accounts of lay people can provide an important basis for interrogating these mean-ings, by challenging the imperatives of neo-liberal rule and opening up some space for considering the possibilities for more democratic forms of rule. Because lay knowledges draw on a highly diverse array of sources (see my response to Patricia's question), they can be used as a basis for challenging what counts as valid descriptions of the social and natural world. As one of the important contemporary languages for describing our world – for explaining both our body make-up and our social differ-ences – genetics is, I believe, a crucial site for questioning what is taken to be natural and normal.

Many people have begun to give thought to the issue of how to increase 'citizens'' participation in wider democratic processes, without reducing this participation to that of consumer. And some of this work concerns decision making in relation to the new genetics. The work of Kerr *et al.*, referred to in my chapter, is based on the use of lay people's accounts as a resource for discussion about the new genetics. Their use of focus groups is an attempt to create an environment conducive to the ex-ploration and expression of people's diverse views, while allowing partic-ipants to make connections between the public and private aspects of their lives. As Kerr *et al.* argue, lay accounts are an important resource in raising questions which are otherwise ignored in policy discussions. The challenge is to create, and legitimise, mechanisms that allow for the direct input of these views into decision making processes. The use of 'citizens' juries' is one possibility. Recently, in Wales there has been an attempt to use 'citizens' juries' to enhance public discussion of and participation in decision making surrounding the introduction of new genetic tech-nologies into health care. The jury was randomly chosen to broadly represent the Welsh population in terms of the major socioeconomic variables. This jury was presented with a question related to genetic testing for predispositions to common disorders, then allowed the opportunity to examine evidence, interrogate expert witnesses, debate the issues and come to a decision. The whole process was facilitated by an experienced moderator (see Dunkerley and Glasner 1998). Although in this case the process was not without its limitations and problems, the 'citizens' jury' approach shows promise in terms of the greater demo-cratisation of decision making in relation to genetics. 'Citizens' juries' have been used for decision making about important public issues in other parts of Britain, as well as in Germany and the USA, with varying degrees of 'success'. I believe much more thought needs to be given to exploring the utility of this mechanism, and other mechanisms, for facilitating the democratisation of policy making. In the area of genetics and public health/medicine, this would include the development of strategies that enhance the input of lay people into decision making about programmes of research and the clinical applications of genetics.

Reference

Dunkerley, D. and Glasner, P. (1998) 'Empowering the public? Citizens' juries and the new genetic technologies', *Critical Public Health*, 8, 3: 181–92.

Question from Janice: Your chapter alludes to the changing social understanding or construction of the notion of 'health', or what it means to be 'healthy' – from, first, the absence of illness such as infectious disease; to, second, individual well-being, as evidenced by, for example, public health campaigns to encourage individuals either to reduce or to give up smoking, or to reorientate their diets towards 'healthy' eating, or to take more exercise; to the present development of 'health' as the absence of genetic 'defect'. Implicit in the requirement of the citizen to be reproductively responsible is the premise that the genetically imper-fect offspring would be better off not having been born. This essentialises the human being as principally embodied, and seems to me to be a collapsing of the classical Cartesian mind–body dualism of modernity, which has traditionally valorised the mind and its rationality over the body. Whereas the body – perfect or imperfect – was principally a receptacle for the rational self, the new genetics appears to privilege the body, free of genetic imperfections, over other aspects of human subjectivity. I'd be interested in your comments regarding this 'inversion'/reversal.

Response: Janice, I'm not sure that I agree that the new genetics has involved an 'inversion' or reversal of the mind–body dualism. It does, however, entail a different conception of the body and of what is required to maintain a 'normal', 'healthy' existence from that evident in earlier regimes of public health. There is still a sense in which the mind is valorised and the body is subject to control by a rational self. The modern public health movement has been centrally concerned with both regulating inter-actions between bodies (e.g. quarantine) and inculcating correct body habits through education. In the nineteenth-century public health reports, such as Chadwick's report, to which I referred, one can find many references to the need to educate people to overcome their supposedly 'unhealthy' habits. The hygienist movement that emerged in the late nine-teenth century was concerned with instilling correct behaviours (i.e. cleanliness) so as to keep the germs at bay. This emphasis has continued up to the present, and is even reflected to some extent in the life-style orientation of contemporary health promotion. However, with the new genetics, the 'owner' of the body is seen to have a somewhat different disposition. They are expected to be less reliant on the experts to control disease and infection and to become more autonomous.

The rhetoric of empowerment is central to the new genetics as it is to the public health more generally: the individual is given the freedom to make an 'informed choice' in decision making. However, as I argued, 'freedom' is compromised by the language of risks and by citizenship responsibilities to others, especially to one's family members and future offspring. The recent development of the notions of 'fetal rights' and 'prenatal abuse' or 'fetal negligence', at least in some (e.g. US) jurisdic-tions (see Merchant 1996), for example, provides a powerful constraint on the exercise of 'free choice'. Nevertheless, at least in rhetoric, the objective is to enhance personal autonomy. The genetic image of the body – as specialised, yet flexible and perfectible – mirrors the contemporary ideal of the self. The rationality of neo-liberalism demands that the indi-vidual seeks constant self-improvement and is capable of adapting to a constantly changing environment. The vision of the perfectible body and the perfectible self, although not new, has come to the fore with the new genetics. Knowing one's own genetic risk and taking rational steps to avoid or minimise risk have become an increasingly central part of being a healthy self. What we have, in effect, is a up-dated version of Social Darwinism. The adaptors survive, the inflexible perish.

Reference

Merchant, J. (1996) 'Biogenetics, artificial procreation, and public policy in the United States and France', *Technology in Society*, 18, 1: 1–15.

Chapter 5

Technology and citizenship

Ian Barns

The renewal of a discourse of active citizenship[1] in western liberal democratic polities in recent years has been in large part a reaction to the ascendancy of neo-liberalism in social policy and its consequent corrosive impact on public life and social institutions (Meredyth 1997; Mouffe 1988). Recent poststructuralist analyses of this renewed civic discourse has been critical of the abstractness of notions of 'civil society', 'citizenship' and the like and has focused on developing more detailed genealogical accounts of the ways in which these and other such notions have functioned within the government of populations (Burchell 1995). In this chapter I'm interested in two rather different features of such discourse. The first is the sometimes explicit, though mostly implicit (and in the case of poststructuralists rather more muted), moral concern which animates much of the critical response to neo-liberalism and the advocacy of active citizenship. Notwithstanding our critical reservations in an academic context about moral discourse, when it comes to public policy issues, those of us who come from a more or less leftist, feminist or social democratic background feel a sense of moral dismay when we observe the effects of neo-liberal social policies on people: the growing inequality of wealth, income and life chances, the increasing surveillance, the dismantling or reconstruction of public institutions as profit making companies, the growing callousness and meanness of public life. We have a perhaps poorly articulated but deeply felt sense of the unfairness of it all, a sense of dismay at the erosion of human dignity and the withdrawal of social rights, especially for the poorest and the most vulnerable. We still believe that government should act for the 'common good' (however difficult that may be to define), providing resources for health, education, welfare and employment generation to enable ordinary people to flourish as individuals and as communities. We still have an intuitive sense of citizenship as a moral practice, of the virtues of being involved in civic issues, of the rightness of fighting developers, cost cutting governments and so on. Yet in the context of postmodern and poststructuralist critiques of modernist grand narratives we find it hard to develop any rational foundation for such moral feelings. Indeed, we are uncomfortable, even suspicious, of normative discourse altogether. We deconstruct the language of morality as a technique of governmentality, ethics as a moral technology (Rose 1990). Thus, despite our moral feelings, in the end we are uncertain as to whether it is possible to talk about citizenship as a moral practice at all. As a consequence, in so far as our responses are typical of academics on the left more generally, by default the language of morality in public life ends up being coopted by conservatives and reactionaries for the cause of moral prohibition, racism and sometimes xenophobic nationalism.

The second feature I want to talk about is the relatively little attention given to technology in the renewed civic discourse, both as a significant factor in the emergence of neo-liberalism and as an important dimension of active citizenship. This relative neglect is quite striking, given the fact that the rise of advanced liberalism as a dominant public policy discourse was at least in part catalysed by the advent of a new generation of information and communication technologies (Hinkson 1993). Clearly, the diffusion of these technologies through economic, political and social life has significantly affected the capacity of governments to control national economies, thus providing a more favourable climate for neo-liberal ideas. New communications technologies have enabled banks and corporations to move capital around the world quickly and in large volumes, and to coordinate production and marketing of products in a more flexible and precise fashion, allowing them to take advantage of competitive opportunities and new niche markets as they arise. New technologies have made possible changes in production processes, which in turn have dramatically altered the nature and availability of work, including the emergence of a global workforce and downward pressures on wages and conditions. The new information and communication technologies are also themselves the consumer goods of globalising culture industries which exert significant pressures on national cultural identities and practices.

The absence of critical reflection in policy debates about the social and cultural significance of technology is also striking when we consider the burgeoning literature on the cultural meanings of new technologies, especially, for example, with respect to the implications of the 'second information age', for self-identity and so on (Poster 1994). Certainly in cultural and communication studies technology has emerged as a central focus for cultural analysis, particularly in terms of the ways in which communication technologies, from television to the emergent cyberspace and the new genetics, are powerful factors in shaping late modern or postmodern identities (Giddens 1991; Jameson 1991).

In this chapter my aim is to apply a constructivist approach to the analysis of technology as a social and cultural phenomenon, an analysis that I hope complements the other chapters in this volume. As Langdon Winner (1997) has recently commented, there is now a broad constructivist consensus amongst historians, philosophers and sociologists of science and technology. However, as Winner says, it is a 'jarring irony' that technological determinism reigns supreme in the new era of dazzling information and communications technology. In the context of public policy debates about technology developments, constructivists face a daunting task in contesting the seeming neutrality and 'technicity' of technological development and rendering visible its character as a social process. At least there is an affinity between constructivist approaches to technology and poststructuralist analyses of neo-liberal governance, particularly in the importance attached to the discursive function of technologies in structuring social life.[2] From a constructivist perspective, poststructuralists develop a more finely structured analysis of the ways in which fields of human activity are constituted within an instrumental rationality which is essentially manipulative in nature. The analysis of governmentalisation highlights the significance of neo-liberalism as not just simply a withdrawal of the state from the supposedly 'free market', but rather as an actually more invasive instrumentalisation and meta-control of social life (Meredyth 1997; Muetzelfeldt 1992).

One of the underlying reasons for the neglect of critical reflection on technology in public policy discourse is the continuing influence of externalist conceptions of technology.[3] Technologies are seen either as tools, morally neutral in themselves, which we use more or less efficiently or more or less badly, or as a larger determining force to which we must adapt or with which we must strive to keep up. Either way, they remain external to the domain of human subjectivity and moral agency (Joerges 1988). What this view lacks is a sense of the constitutive importance of technologies: that technologies are not external to us, but are implicated in the ongoing processes of self-construction. As Langdon Winner has pointed out, technologies are not merely tools that we use instrumentally. They are, more deeply, 'forms of life' such that as we incorporate them into our lives they subtly change our relationships with the world, our sense of community and even more deeply our own sense of self-identity and embodiment:

> As they become woven into the texture of everyday existence, the devices, techniques, and systems we adopt shed their tool-like qualities to become part of our very humanity. In an important sense we become the beings who work on assembly lines, who talk on telephones, who do our figuring on pocket calculators, who eat processed foods, who clean our homes with powerful chemicals.
>
> (Winner 1986b: 13)

A constructivist approach to technology probes beneath the instrumental meanings of technology, including questions of environmental impacts or health and safety, and even implications for the distribution of information, wealth and power. It develops an interpretative exploration of the ways in which technologies are involved in reshaping the spaces and discourses of social life and in the ongoing construction of subjectivity. It analyses the ways in which the technologies embodied in diverse artefacts, everyday stocks of technical know-how, administrative rules, large-scale systems, technical experts and so on are interpreted or articulated within the domain of social practices, and how they are involved in the formation of personal and civic identity.

In this chapter, then, I want to consider in broad terms how the diffusion of modern/late modern technologies affects the kind of people we are, how it enters into our formation as moral agents and what this means for the project of recovering ideas of active citizenship and civil society. As I've already noted, most modernist discourse still assumes that technological innovation is generally a progressive or emancipatory force, notwithstanding concerns about the 'ethical dilemmas' posed by the new technologies of genetics and information technology. Despite fears that pornography and images of violence on the Internet might harm impressionable young people, or that genetic technologies might lead to a brave new world of designer people, or that plant biotechnologies might lead to a concentration of genetic resources in the hands of transnational agribusinesses, few participants in public debates seriously question the ultimately progressive direction of continuing technological innovation. It just needs to be better regulated, or directed in democratic and sustainable directions.

By contrast, a central theme in postmodernist analyses of rapidly changing media technologies is that the effect of such technologies has been to undermine, decentre, fragment and externalise the humanist self assumed by modernist political creeds: liberal democratic, social democratic, civic republican or otherwise (Kroker 1992). The best-known example of such postmodern critique, Donna Haraway's cyborg manifesto (Haraway 1987, 1991b) proclaims a radical break with the framework of enlightenment humanism, repudiating a return to a premodern arcadia and, instead, subversively embracing a posthumanist 'cyborg' identity. What isn't clear is whether citizenship would mean much to a posthumanist cyborg.

However, the trouble with much of this literature is that despite its scornful dismissal of an abstract modernism, its own abstractness and rhetorical overstatement also mystifies and distorts the complex ways in which contemporary technologies are involved in forming ordinary people in the ordinariness of everyday life. The fascination with cutting-edge technologies, especially cyberspace, and with science fiction representations of human existence in a world of pervasive technologies means that the myriad ways in which ordinary people continue to form relationships and participate more or less meaningfully in a technologically mediated civic life are not taken seriously. We are not all cyborgs; we are not routinely confronted by a nature turned 'alien' by the logic of domination. Furthermore, as Andrew Ross has commented, if it overstates the all-encompassing power of 'technoculture' in reaction to modernist complacency, postmodern critique can lead to a deep sense of powerlessness and pessimism (Penley and Ross 1991).

In making sense of technology we should thus not allow grand oracular celebration or denunciations of cyberculture to silence the diverse meanings of technology in the contexts of our everyday, embodied ordinariness. Vivian Sobchak's response to Baudrillard's enthusiasm for the 'techno-erotic' in J.G. Ballard's *Crash* should give us heart. Sobchak observes ironically that 'Indeed, writing about *Crash*, the lived-body sitting at Baudrillard's desk must have forgotten itself to celebrate, instead, "a body with neither organs nor organ pleasures, entirely dominated by gash marks, cut-outs, and technical scars".' She goes on to talk about her own pain and fear in her experience of cancer, commenting wryly:

> there is nothing like a little pain to bring us back to our senses, nothing like a real (not imagined) mark or wound to counter the romanticism and fantasies of techno-sexual transcendence that characterizes so much of the current discourse on the techno-body that is thought to occupy the cyberspaces of post-modernity ... Thus, sharp pain, dull aches and numbness (which after all, is not not-feeling, but feeling of not-feeling), the cold touch of technology on my flesh, were distractions from my erotic possibilities, and not, as Baudrillard would have it, erotically distracting.
>
> (Sobchak 1995: 205–14)

What I want to do, then, is to try to capture something of the complexity and ambiguity of continuing technological develop-ments, to do justice both to the ordinary, everyday life-world experience of technological practice as well as to the deeper cultural transformation associated with the rapid diffusion of late modern technologies. Following Brian Fay's (1987) approach to the inter-pretation of social practices, I shall suggest that we need to attend to the meanings of technology in our social practices at three levels: first, the primary level of life-world experience, of the diverse ways in which we experience, apply, interpret and represent the tech-nologies that become part of our lives and how such practices affect subjectivity, self-identity and social relations; second, the level of the larger political economy of technoeconomic systems, within which our everyday practices are embedded and which thus consti-tute the material, political and symbolic order of our lives; and third, the epistemological framework which underlies and is expressed through technological innovation and diffusion, what Stephen Hill (1988) calls the cultural grammar of technology and what we are describing in this book in terms of 'rationalities of rule'. If we approach technologies in terms of these three levels we may be better able to recognise the ambiguous and complex ways in which they are involved in the shaping of moral agency: through the some-times consumerist, sometimes improvisory, sometimes subversive life-world adaptations of technology; through the operation of the larger political forces directing the choice, design, representation and regulation of technologies in ways that expand markets, increase profits, open up new commodities and centralise strategic control over social life; and through the continuing articulation of the modernist cultural project of an instrumental control of the world (and more specifically through liberal and neo-liberal forms of governance).

My argument is that, notwithstanding the flexibility of everyday technological practices and the enhancement of moral agency that they make possible, at a deeper level the continuing trajectory of technological change is towards a continuing commodification and instrumentalisation of human life, partly because of the strategic interests of capital, but more profoundly because of the cultural grammar that technological innovation expresses. In other words, the most fundamental significance of contemporary technology is as a reading or a construction of the world, not just 'intellectually' but practically. In the end, though, it is a reading/construction which is fundamentally self-contradictory inasmuch as, although it arises out of and is sustained by humanist promise of self-empowerment, yet even as it is realised in the practical circumstances of social life it reconstructs human experience and subjectivity itself as the stuff of instrumental control. Ultimately, the modernist project of humanising or regulating modern technology is incoherent and self-defeating. Yet so also is the rhetoric of a posthumanism which embraces the dissolution of the humanist self. Rather, I want to suggest that the reading of the world expressed through modern technologies is fundamentally a misreading which may distort and attenuate but never extinguish the everyday experience of moral agency. Following Charles Taylor (1989), I shall argue that the civic humanist advocacy of active citizenship, despite its abstractness and failure to recognise the incorporation of the language of citizenship within the discourse of neo-liberal discourse, none the less points to the need for a recovery of moral ontology, not just at the level of abstract philosophy but at the level of technological practice.

Making sense of technology

Technology in the context of everyday practices

First, in trying to make sense of technology we need to focus on what Albert Borgmann (1984) calls the 'foreground' of technology: our everyday practical engagement with the diversity of technological devices, procedures and systems that inhabit our worlds. As Borgmann comments, it is easy to discuss technology abstractly, focusing our attention on the more abstract techno-logical systems and structures. In so doing we can easily reify technology, treating it as a force which impinges upon our lives from outside. Instead, we need to attend to the dialectical nature of technologies in the practices of everyday life (Drengson 1995): both the ways in which people give shape and meaning to technologies in their everyday practices and, conversely, the ways in which as they are taken up in people's lives they may subtly and profoundly reshape both life world and people (Silverstone 1989).

Brian Wynne (1988) has argued that we need to recognise the 'unruliness' and indeterminate open-ness of complex technological devices and systems. The context of Wynne's argument was a discussion of how to make sense of such accidents as the Challenger disaster and the explosion in the ICI plant at Bhopal, India in the 1980s. Rather than viewing technological accidents as simply the result of aberrant human carelessness or corruption in what would otherwise normally be an orderly, rule-governed activity, Wynne suggests that such events enable us to glimpse the 'normal' unruliness, adaptation, corner-cutting and so on which take place all the time in the operation of technological devices and systems, from domestic life to high-tech factories. In other words, within our life-world practices, we, from home dwellers to workers in high-tech factories, are continually making judgements and bending the rules, sometimes taking risks and being careless. Wynne suggests that even in the most technologically complex and sophisticated environments, the exercise of human practical judgement consti-tutes the irreplaceable basis for the way technologies work.

In her book, *In the Age of the Smart Machine,* Shoshanna Zuboff (1988) provides a wonderful example of the ways in which indus-trial technologies are contextualised and adapted within life-world practices. Zuboff describes a high-tech pulp mill where access between the control room and a snack area was regulated by two automatic sliding doors. The operation of the doors was designed in such a way as to prevent hot air from the plant operations entering the control room.

> This is not what most men do when they move from the control room out into the bleach plant. They step through the inner door, but they do not wait for that door to seal behind

them before opening the second door. Instead, they force their fingertips through the rubber seal down the middle of the outer door and, with a mighty heft of their shoulders, pry open the seam and wrench the door apart. Hour after hour, shift after shift, week after week, too many men pit the strength in their arms and shoulders against the electronic mechanism that controls the doors. Three years after the construction of the sleek, glittering glass bubble, the outer door no longer closes tightly.

(Zuboff 1988: 21)

This seemingly incidental (mis)use of a technological device illuminates the often unruly and improvisory ways in which technologies get adapted and interpreted within people's lives. Although devices, systems and procedures have been designed by planners, engineers and policy makers with certain rule-governed practices in mind, there is still considerable openness and flexibility in terms of how they are used and what they are used for. We can extend this observation to say that there is, more generally, an inherent indeterminacy or unpredictability as to what the social meanings of technologies will be at the level of life-world practice, and that such meanings can only be discovered by an interpretative investigation of the diverse ways in which technologies are actually used and contextualised in domestic, occupational and social environments.

In recent years there have been many such interpretative studies of the ways in which particular technologies have been adapted within specific life-world situations. Examples include the work of Silverstone *et al.* analysing the social meanings of 'consuming technologies' (Silverstone and Hirsch 1992), Cynthia Cockburn on the gender meanings that become attached to domestic technology devices such as microwave ovens (Cockburn 1992; Cockburn and Furst-Dilic 1994) and Sherry Turkle's exploration of the experiences of people at the computer 'interface' (Turkle 1984, 1995). As Morley and Silverstone (1990: 32) have commented about television as a domestic technology:

television's meanings, that is the meanings of both texts and technologies, have to be understood as emergent properties of contextualised audience practices. These practices have to be seen as situated within the facilitating and constraining microsocial environments of family and household interaction.

While it is true, though, that the meanings of technologies are significantly determined by what people make of them in the context of everyday practices, conversely it is also true that the diffusion of technologies will often subtly transform social practices, identities and relationships. As already mentioned earlier in this chapter, Langdon Winner has observed that as we adopt new devices, procedures and systems, often for the pursuit of existing practical and symbolic purposes, their incorporation will bring about often unforeseen and unintended changes in social life, in the way we relate to each other and to our natural environment and in the languages we employ. Often the most dramatic examples come from the introduction of industrial technologies into less-developed societies. For example, in *Democracy and Technology*, Richard Sclove (1995) describes the surprising social effects resulting from the simple introduction of piped running water into a Spanish village which had hitherto depended on a single village well for its water:

> Arduous tasks were rendered technologically superfluous, but village social life unexpectedly changed. The public fountain and washbasin, once scenes of vigorous social interaction, became nearly deserted. Men began losing their sense of famil-iarity with the children and the donkeys that had once helped them to haul water. Women stopped congregating at the wash-basin to intermix their scrubbing with politically empowering gossip about men and village life. In hindsight, the installation of running water helped break down the Ibiecans' strong bonds – with one another, with their animals, and with the land – that had knit them together as a community.
>
> (Ibid.: 3)

Commenting on the social transformation accompanying the diffusion of the automobile, Winner (1986b: 9) observes:

> In hindsight the situation is clear to everyone. Individual habits, perceptions, concepts of self, ideas of space and time, social relationships, and moral and political boundaries have all been powerfully restructured in the course of modern technological development. What is fascinating about this process is that soci-eties involved in it have quickly altered some of the fundamental terms of human life without appearing to do so.

A more specific application of Winner's general comment on 'automobility' as a form of life is provided by Gyorgy Scrinis's (1997) reflections on the phenomenon of 'road rage'. Whilst recognising the wider changes in social life that prompt people to act ever more aggressively to others on the road, Scrinis comments that 'the source of this behaviour can ultimately be traced back to the way the car so thoroughly transforms the way in which the driver engages with the world when he (or she) is behind the wheel'. He goes on to talk about the compression of our experience of space and time and the encapsulation of the driver in an all-encompassing technological environment with a much more limited engagement with the world outside:

> In these ways the car profoundly mediates and shapes the driver's way of encountering the world. Drivers come to confront each other not as vulnerable, mortal all-too-human beings, but as human–machine hybrids. Social relations between people begin to take the form of instrumental relations between machines.
>
> (Ibid.: A15)

The automobile is an old, now familiar technology and we are more or less familiar with the range of cultural meanings and the relationships with people, streets and the natural environment that it tends to promote. We have also had over forty years of mass broadcasting, and the experience of television and its associated forms of life and subjectivities have likewise been explored intensively. Contemporary interest, however, is now focused on the new media, on life in cyberspace, and the experience of networking and interactivity (Poster 1994; Featherstone and Burrows 1995; Loader 1997; Aronowitz *et al.* 1996).

In this section I'm suggesting that we need to focus initially on everyday practice to understand the various ways in which specific technologies are interpreted by particular people and communities, notwithstanding their specific design characteristics and technical-functional logic and purposes. On the one hand, such technologies will allow a finite range of possible applications. How they are actually interpreted will depend a great deal on people's life-world interests, how technologies are represented, particularly in commercial advertising, but also through the interpretative influence of experts, regulators and early adaptors. Advertising plays a crucial role in imaginatively locating new devices within life-world possibilities; for example, the ways in which a mobile phone might serve practical and symbolic purposes within a cosmopolitan lifestyle. Yet, as I've suggested above, the ways in which such possibilities are taken up and the kinds of 'worlds' that emerge cannot easily be predicted. They are, as Winner comments, emergent realities.

Technoeconomic systems

The experiences and practices of everyday life are always embedded within larger and increasingly complex interconnected systems or structures. To be sure, most of us are only vaguely aware of how such background systems work and how our lives depend upon them, particularly at the level of the complex technologies which frame and sustain our lives. David Lodge (1989: 269) nicely captures this unreflective embeddedness in his novel, *Nice Work*. As she flies off to Hamburg with the factory manager, Vic, Robyn Penrose, the academic specialising in nineteenth-century industrial novels, looks down upon the streets and cities of England:

> Sunlight flooded the cabin as the plane changed course. It was a bright, clear morning. Robyn looked out of the window as England slid slowly beneath them: cities and towns, their street plans like printed circuits, scattered over a mosaic of tiny fields, connected by thin wires of railways and motorways. Hard to imagine at this height all the noise and commotion going on down there. Factories, shops, offices, schools, beginning the working day. People crammed into rush hour buses and trains, or sitting at the wheels of their cars in traffic jams, or washing up breakfast things in the kitchens of pebble dashed semis. All inhabiting their own little worlds, oblivious of how they fitted into the total picture. The housewife, switching on her electric kettle to make another cup of tea, gave no thought to the immense complex of operations that made that simple action possible: the building and maintenance of the power station that produced the electricity, the mining of coal or pumping of oil to fuel the generators, the laying of miles of cable to carry the current to her house, the digging and smelting of and milling of ore or bauxite into sheets of steel or aluminium, the cutting and pressing and welding of the metal into the kettle's shell, spout and handle, the assembly of these parts with scores of

other components – coils, screws, nuts, bolts, washers, rivets, wires, springs, rubber insulation, plastic trimmings; then the packaging of the kettle, the advertising of the kettle, the marketing of the kettle to wholesale and retail outlets, the transportation of the kettle to warehouses and shops, the calculation of its price, and the distribution of its added value between all the myriad people and agencies concerned in its production and circulation. The housewife gave no thought to all this as she switched on her kettle.

Making sense of large-scale technological systems is an important challenge for constructivist approaches to technology. As Thomas Misa (1988) has noted, the more abstract the level of analysis, the greater the tendency towards a technological determinism which reifies the supposedly autonomous logic of the system. However, most constructivist studies of development of technological systems, such as the work of Bijker *et al.* (1986), emphasise their socially constructed character. Winner, for example, draws our attention to the political significance of the ways in which technological systems are designed. Such systems are, he claims, ways of building order in the world, similar to legislation in constructing a more or less enduring institutional framework within which we live our lives:

> The things we call 'technologies' are ways of building order in our world. Many technical devices and systems important in everyday life contain possibilities for many different ways of ordering human activity. Consciously or unconsciously, deliberately or inadvertently, societies choose structures for technologies that influence how people are going to work, communicate, travel, consume, and so forth over a very long time. In the processes by which structuring decisions are made, different people are situated differently and possess unequal degrees of power as well as unequal levels of awareness. By far the greatest latitude of choice exists the very first time a particular instrument, system, or technique is introduced. Because choices tend to become strongly fixed in material equipment, economic investment, and social habit, the original flexibility vanishes for all practical purposes once the initial commitments are made. In that sense technological innovations are similar to legislative acts or political foundings that

establish a framework for public order that will endure over many generations. For that reason the same careful attention one would give to the rules, roles, and relationships of politics must also be given to such things as the building of highways, the creation of television networks, and the tailoring of seemingly insignificant features of new machines. The issues that divide or unite people in society are settled not only in the institutions and practices of politics proper, but also, and less obviously, in tangible arrangement of steel and concrete, wires and semiconductors, nuts and bolts.

(Winner 1986b: 28)

Unfortunately, the inherently political nature of technological systems is still poorly recognised within a public discourse which focuses on technical efficiency, productivity and economic competitiveness (Winner 1997). Our existing technological systems, ranging from urban transport systems to energy generation and transmission systems to less obviously 'technological' administrative and regulatory systems, all continue to embody, and perhaps reinforce, the political purposes which they were consciously or unconsciously designed to serve. Also, their material and institutional objectification makes it difficult to restructure them in any fundamental way. On the other hand, the creation of new technological systems, such as the so-called information superhighway does provide a brief window of opportunity for the intentional shaping of such a system around basic democratic ideals (Mathews 1989).

In recent years there has been much discussion about changing techno-economic paradigms (Dosi 1982), particularly in terms of long waves of technological change (Perez 1983) or a shift from Fordism to post-Fordism. (Amin 1994). It has been the latter, originating from the work of the French 'regulation school' (Aglietta 1987) which has been most influential in the analysis of fundamental shifts in capitalist societies associated with radical technological innovations. According to this approach, 'Fordism' describes an economic and institutional order that provides the regulatory or control framework for a production system which is itself built upon the core technologies of mass production (Roobeek 1987). Despite the fact that the model posits that within a Fordist paradigm the logic of mass production is reflected in wider political and administrative systems as well as in educational and cultural life, the analysis is only partially deterministic. Roobeek, for example, argues that the establishment of a Fordist paradigm in various nation-states between 1920 and 1960 involved significant national differences.

According to this view, the growing multilevel crisis of Fordism which emerged in the 1970s provided the stimulus for the introduction of emerging information technologies, biotechnologies and advanced materials technologies, in the hope that they would overcome the problems of productivity, declining markets and the like. Instead, they provided the catalyst for a paradigmatic shift in production systems, a shift away from high-volume, standardised mass production towards greater flexible specialisation in the production of high-quality customised goods for more diverse niche markets. These post-Fordist developments in core production processes have in turn created the need for a very different economic and institutional order and have contributed to a significant shift in social attitudes and cultural expectations. Such an analysis also suggests an interesting connection between changes in production systems and the emergence of a more fragmented culture of post-modernity (Harvey 1989).

Some analysts, such as the Australian John Mathews, argued that the emergence of new production systems created a 'window of opportunity' for democratic participation in the design of new social and political institutions. In *Age of Democracy,* Mathews (1989) argued that the break-up of the old Fordist paradigm presented a challenge and opportunity for the reconstruction of social democracy in terms of a programme of 'associative democracy' which drew upon the heritage of the labour movement and the energies of the new social movements.

Although the idea of a transition from Fordism to post-Fordism was embraced by some in the early 1990s, most notably those associated with the journal *Marxism Today*, its optimistic view that new forms of capitalist production would open up possibilities for a more cooperative and democratic relationship between capital and labour were widely criticised (Jessop 1990; Fieldes and Bramble 1992; Hirst and Zeitlin 1991). Critics such as Simon Clarke (1990) argued that, far from signifying a paradigmatic shift in capitalist economic production, the key developments were not those of the introduction of new technologies, but the initiation of restructuring processes by a globalising capitalism that would overcome the barriers of labour resistance.

Whilst the ideas of post-Fordism have been taken up in various ways, for example by David Harvey (1989) in *The Condition of Postmodernity,* the focus of critical attention has shifted to other structural changes in capitalism, such as the processes of globalisation (Hirst and Thompson 1996), 'risk society' (Beck 1992), the 'network society' (Castells 1997) and what Lash and Urry (1994) call 'reflexive accumulation', by which they mean the central importance of knowledge-intensive production activities. Nevertheless, there is a general recognition that we do live in a time of deeper structural change in technoeconomic systems, change that is particularly associated with the diffusion of information and communication technologies. The informationalisation of economic life has in turn been the catalyst for what are perhaps only the beginnings of a broader transformation of political institutions and social and cultural life.

The cultural frame of modern technology

The third level that needs to be considered in making sense of the technologies of everyday life is that of the 'cultural frame' which lies behind them and which they 'realise' in material and organisational forms. There are many who argue that all that lies 'behind' technological development is the power of globalising capitalism. For example, Frederic Jameson (1991: 36) asserts:

> our faulty representations of some immense communication and computer network are themselves but a distorted figuration of something even deeper, namely the whole world system of a present day multinational capitalism. The technology of contemporary society is therefore mesmerizing and fascinating not so much in its own right but because it seems to offer some privileged representational shorthand for grasping a network of power and control even more difficult for our minds and imagination to grasp: the whole new decentred global network of the third stage of capital itself.

Yet the 'whole system of multinational capitalism' and the technoeconomic systems through which it is mediated is itself located within a taken-for-granted epistemological and ontological framework which we describe broadly in terms of modernity, enlightenment reason or instrumental rationality (Feenberg 1992;

Pippin 1995). I don't wish to discuss this background cultural frame in any detail. My interest is in the ways in which it is articulated or 'materialised' through the ongoing processes of specific technological developments. That is to say, I'm interested in the ways in which contemporary technologies involve a particular reading of the world, or better: an active construction of the world in terms of ongoing instrumental control. I'm suggesting that as our everyday practices are continually reconstructed in terms of the implicit cultural logic of devices, systems, organisational rationalities, we learn to read the world, other people and ultimately ourselves in terms of an instrumentalist epistemology, and more significantly to experience the fate of its central binaries: between self and other, subject and object, means and ends.

This level of analysis is associated in particular with Heidegger's (1977) notion of technology as the culmination of that western metaphysical tradition which constitutes nature as 'standing reserve', with Jacques Ellul's (1964) analysis of modern society in terms of the ongoing expression of '*la technique*', and more recently Albert Borgmann's (1984) analysis of the 'device paradigm'. What is distinctive about this analysis is that it goes beyond mainstream sociological analyses of the abstract processes of rationalisation and disenchantment to examine the ways in which such processes are expressed in and through technologically mediated systems and life-world practices. It suggests that we need to learn to decipher our technologies, to probe beneath their functional and practical uses and even the politicoeconomic purposes they may have been designed to serve, to grasp the underlying cultural 'code' that they express.

What is particularly significant here is that the technological objectification of the cultural project of an instrumental control of nature, once a utopian dream, realises unrecognised and hitherto implicit meanings of that project. As well as being a cultural project, technology is also a cultural experiment. In *The Tragedy of Technology,* Stephen Hill (1988) develops this theme in terms of the analysis of technology as a language. Specific technologies are 'cultural texts' and we know how to make sense of these 'texts' because we are familiar with the instrumentalist 'cultural grammar' which underlies them. We thus need to probe behind the immediate technical knowledge required in our engagement with technologies to explicate their background cultural grammar (ibid.: 43). In this perspective:

Contemporary technology is therefore not merely a set of tools or artefacts that assume meaning according to a wider cultural frame of values and assumptions. Indeed, contemporary technology symbolises the frame itself, within which our cultural possibilities are cast and played out – a frame that industrial society willingly embraced when instrumental logic was welcomed as master rather than as servant to social arrangements.

(Ibid.: 56)

The claim that our lives are increasingly embedded within, 'enframed' by, an epistemology, a metaphysic, of instrumental rationality which increasingly pervades social, economic and political life, mediated through the commodifying purposes of late modern capitalism still seems entirely implausible to most citizens of liberal democratic societies. Or perhaps, more accurately, it remains repressed, an unsettling, unconscious anxiety that is explored not in public policy debate but in popular science fiction. In public life at least, the notion of technological enframement seems to be directly contradicted by the promise that new technologies will extend our personal autonomy and enrich our sociality. Certainly within mainstream policy discourse, the language of politics and democracy, still seems to enframe technology and not the other way around.

In a modernist perspective, then, the novelty of, and human possibilities opened up by, ongoing technological developments continue to fascinate us and at times alarm us, particularly in areas of biomedical science and molecular genetics. With the remarkable, Promethean human genome project and its central goal of disclosing the genetic basis of human differences, there is an uneasy recognition that such developments might mean a rethinking of the nature and basis of human identity. The typical response is one of anxiety about the potential threat to human rights and a rhetorical concern about the dehumanising effects of technology. In relation to the new genetics there is anxiety about designing people – the possibility of designer babies, etc. Yet this discourse assumes a genetic essentialism which does not address the more complex and subtle ways in which technological artefacts, procedures and systems reshape our identities. By and large there is a continuing inability to recognise the cultural frame of instrumentalism which lies behind such techniques and which already more deeply reconstitutes human subjectivity and identity in instrumentalist terms.[4]

This modernist, instrumentalist discourse masks not only the background horizon of instrumentalism within which technological innovation takes place, but also the processes of linguistic transformation by which the humanist language of democracy, justice, rights becomes effectively redefined in technological terms. In the view of Peter Emberley (1989: 744–5)

> the global network which increasingly constitutes the context of our lives is mobilized by technologies which displace the intelligibility and effectiveness of our traditional moral and political categories. We are experiencing an alteration of what we have taken phenomena to be and to mean within an emerging environment of electronic transmissions of information, data-processing industries, satellite technology, global telecommunications, recombinant genetic microbiology, and social cybernetics. These technologies are indicative of a significant alteration and have created an environment where the bases of our moral and political terms – the 'Euclidean' notions of space (enclosure and exclusion) and time (succession and duration) which constituted the human experience of sequentiality, causality, continuity, have lost their ordering power.

Yet this technologising takes place not only through the ways in which specific devices and 'hardware' systems function as 'discourse', but also through the pervasive shift within public policy and professional discourses and practices. In this perspective a neo-liberal public policy framework is an expression of the ongoing spread of '*la technique*', manifested in the restructuring of the whole range of micro-practices of education, health and welfare delivery. We experience what Leslie Thiele (1995: 197) in his commentary on Heidegger's concept of technology calls the 'Midas touch' of technology:

> Technology has a Midas touch and a particularly contagious one at that. Everything with which it comes in contact becomes uniformly subsumed into a framework of efficiently exploited resources. Indeed, technology reconfigures human society itself to accommodate the exigencies of its furthest extensions and intrusions.

John Hinkson (1993) has developed a similar argument about the connection between neo-liberal public policy and the epistemological significance of contemporary technologies. In his notion of a 'postmodern market' Hinkson wants to describe a fundamental shift in the meanings of economic and political processes associated with new communication technologies: a shift that has not been adequately recognised even by regulation theorists such as Aglietta who do not appreciate the 'cultural break' entailed by new technologies: 'a framing of the economy by processes which change its basic character and meaning'.

Contemporary technologies and the crisis of the humanist self

I want to turn now to the broader question of how our engagement with contemporary technologies affects our constitution as selves or moral agents. As I've already noted, notwithstanding the explosion of interest in the relationship between identity and technology amongst postmodern writers, the dominant public discourse continues to be that of an essentially optimistic liberal instrumentalism. New technologies are viewed largely as a prosthetic enhancement of human capabilities.

In postmodern reflection there is a much greater recognition of the more radical implications of contemporary technologies for the humanist self. Much of this arises out of the fragmenting, decentring effects of the diffusion of new media and information technologies (Gergen 1991). As Grodin and Lindlof (1996: 4) comment:

> Mediated communication enables us to encounter many diverse people representing different social enclaves and ethnic or religious backgrounds. In this way, it challenges the validity of singular perspectives and calls into question the hegemony of rational choice and the belief in one truth or rational judgement. Self becomes multivocal as we carry a number of voices with us. Individuals, then, may find that they no longer have a central core with which to evaluate and act, but instead find themselves 'decentred'. Decentredness is also linked to a sense of dislocation, not only in the sense of not being strictly tied to physical place because of mediated opportunities but also in the way self may be mobilised and dispersed.

As this statement suggests, the new communications technologies are implicated in the more radical commodification of social life and social identity, not only of goods and services, but more deeply of experience and subjectivity. Bill Nicholls comments:

> Just as the mechanical reproduction of copies revealed the power of industrial capitalism to reorganise and reassemble the world around us, rendering it as commodity art, the automated intelligence of chips reveals the power of post industrial capitalism to simulate and replace the world around us, rendering not only that exterior realm but also interior ones of consciousness, intelligence, thought and intersubjectivity as commodity experience.
>
> (Quoted in Foster 1996: 278)

The experience of decentredness, fragmentation and commodification of self-hood is reflected in postmodern/poststructuralist critiques of modernist/humanist accounts of the self. Arthur Kroker discusses this in terms of 'the possessed individual' as distinct from the 'possessive individual' of liberal humanism. Discussing contemporary French postmodern writers in terms of their account of technological society Kroker (1992: 13) writes:

> What we witness in contemporary French discourse is a report, all the more uncensored for its theoretical, yet cynical, innocence of its entrapment in the language of technology, of the fate of subjectivity in the postmodern condition, that is, the age when the will to technique achieves its aestheticized point of excess.

The consequence of the deconstruction of the humanist self under the condition of technology, though, is to reveal even our deepest notions of personal freedom and individual autonomy to be 'moral technologies', forms by which regulatory power is expressed within the interstices of everyday life (Rose 1990).

The 'posthumanist' fragmentation and deconstruction of the western (masculinist) humanist self has been enthusiastically, or perhaps defiantly, embraced by some, primarily because of the opportunities it seems to provide to subvert the long-standing dualisms of the enlightenment, particularly between mind and body. The most notable example is Haraway's (1987) cyborg manifesto, in which she urges us to embrace the subversive possibilities within the 'belly of the beast' of late modern capitalist technoculture, rather than by seeking an ecofeminist alternative.

However, such acceptance of postmodern technology as the ultimate frame, however subversively, threatens to undermine the emancipatory promise of a posthumanism altogether and lead to something altogether less hopeful. As John Knight (1995: 33) comments in his contribution to a collection of essays on postmodernism and education:

> Let us suppose, as I fear, that there is a new synthesis of biology, psychology, sociology. We may indeed then have a thorough understanding of 'human nature', a new and effective technology of behaviour, a posthuman constructing indeed. It might also indeed be consonant in its theory and practice with emergent corporatist forms of posteducation. But it would hardly support either the various humanisms of the past or the anti-humanisms of poststructuralism.

The mirage of enlightenment or the recovery of moral ontology

An alternative postmodern response to the technologising and/or deconstruction of the humanist self is to open up the question of the ontological grounding of the self. As Bauman notes, the contemporary instrumentalising of the self through various forms of technological enframing has its roots in the disenchantment of the world more generally. Bauman (1992: xi) outlines the cultural logic of disenchantment as follows:

> as nature became progressively 'de-animated' humans grew increasingly 'naturalized' so that their subjectivity, the primeval 'given-ness' of their existence could be denied and they themselves could be made hospitable for instrumental meanings; they came to be like timber and waterways rather than like forests and lakes. Their disenchantment, like that of the world as a whole, stemmed from the encounter between the designing posture and the strategy of instrumental rationality.

Of course, when there was a confidence in the 'primeval given-ness' of the knowing (humanist) self, the disenchantment of the world and the associated project of instrumental control meant human emancipation and empowerment. As the fundamental ontological contradiction of this humanist project becomes more clearly evident, not just in philosophical terms but through the instrumentalising of the human practice and experience, the critical challenge is one of a reappraisal of disenchantment, a reconsideration of the ontological groundings of self-hood and moral agency. In other words, if our existence as selves, as moral agents, is not 'primevally given', but is dependent upon wider and deeper sources, the question of what those sources are becomes sharper and more urgent. We need to ask the more 'metaphysical' question: What kind of world is it that at least makes possible the emergence of personal and moral existence?

This is the task that Charles Taylor (1989) addresses in *Sources of the Self*. Whilst rejecting any form of essentialism and recognising the narratively constructed nature of the self, Taylor argues that to be a self necessarily assumes some kind of moral orientation or moral ontology. To be a self, he suggests, is to be in moral space, to indwell a moral framework. A moral framework is not something we may or may not choose to have (thus presupposing the independent priority of our selfhood); rather it is presupposed or implicit in becoming and being a self:

> Frameworks provide the background, explicit or implicit, for our moral judgements, intuitions or reactions . . . To articulate a framework is to explicate what makes sense of our moral responses. That is, when we try to spell out what it is that we presuppose when we judge that a certain form of life is truly worthwhile, or place our dignity in a certain achievement or status, or define our moral obligations in a certain manner, we find ourselves articulating inter alia what I have been calling here 'frameworks'.
>
> (Ibid.: 26)

Like other 'communitarian' social philosophers, Taylor argues that the articulation of moral ontology is not primarily a theoretical task, but one of practical reason. That is to say, instead of privileging theory and 'foundations' (or conversely, deconstructing them), we need to focus on social practice in an alternative paradigm of rationality.[5] Or as Taylor puts it elsewhere, we need to reassert the primacy of 'engaged agency' (i.e. 'embodied in a culture, a form of life, a "world" of involvements') rather than 'disengaged agency' (Taylor 1993).

It is only towards the end of *Sources of the Self*, however, that Taylor makes explicit, albeit only partially and briefly, his view that the deepest spiritual sources of the modern self are articulated in and through the Christian tradition (Skinner 1994; Morgan 1994). By this he means not just in the sense of Christianity as a subjectively held belief system, as 'ideas' about God, but as a tradition of practice whose apperception of reality 'grounds' or makes sense of our deepest moral intuitions.

Taylor clearly recognised the difficulties he would face in arguing his Christian, theistic case. More broadly, however, his focus on moral ontology does reflect, perhaps, a 'postsecular turn', an exploration of the possibilities of re-enchantment as the necessary basis for remaining human. For example, Bauman (1992: x) also talks about 're-enchantment':

All in all, postmodernity can be seen as restoring to the world what modernity, presumptuously, has taken away; as a re-enchantment of the world that modernity tried hard to disenchant. It is modern artifice that has been dismantled; the modern conceit of meaning-legislating reason that has been exposed, condemned and put to shame.

Taylor's argument for the recovery of moral ontology and of practical rationality is directed against the pervasive dominance of a naturalistic view of the world which, he argues, increasingly cuts us off from the background, historical moral sources of the modern self. Yet although much of his attention in *Sources of the Self* is directed against instrumentalism as an epistemology, he gives relatively little attention to the question of technology and what a renewed practical rationality might mean in relation to both the dominant cultural frame of contemporary technology and the possible reframing of 'technology' itself as an integral part of 'practice'.

Albert Borgmann (1992) attempts such a task in *Crossing the Postmodern Divide*. He describes the cultural meaning of contemporary technologies in terms of a 'hypermodernity' which, whilst simulating and reconstructing the materiality of our lives, abstracts us more and more from the practices of material 'engagement'. He argues that we need to resist hyperreality by the development of a 'postmodern realism', based not on the attempts to grasp the real through abstract scientific reason, but through an engagement which recovers a sense of the 'focal-ness' of 'things' (as distinct from 'devices' or commodities). Borgmann illustrates this by an account of the specific everyday, civic, festal and religious life of his home town of Missoula in Montana.

Borgmann's account of postmodern realism might easily be dismissed as the complacent utterances of a comfortable American academic removed from the harsh 'postmodern realities' of those who experience the down side of a globalising capitalism. Whilst such a reaction is, I suspect, at least partly justified, none the less I believe that Borgmann does help us to see the ways in which we might live more humanly within our increasing technologised world.

Technology, moral agency and citizenship

The purpose of this extended discussion of how we might think about the cultural meanings of contemporary technology, particularly in relation to constructions of the self, has been to answer the question of what are the implications of contemporary technological developments for attempts to renew the practice of active citizenship. I have tried to answer this question, not by focusing on particular technologies, informational, biomedical or organisational, but rather by outlining an interpretative approach to technology which encompasses the ambiguous and indeterminate possibilities of everyday practices, the institutional context of the techno-economic systems of late modern capitalism, and the deeper cultural frame of 'la technique'. My argument has been that the deepest significance of contemporary technology is that it realises a project of instrumental control which radically undermines the assumptions of the western humanist account of the self. Thus to remain and to flourish as free, personal, moral agents, to maintain the conditions of human dignity, justice, freedom, democracy and the like, requires not just simply the reassertion of popular control over technology. More deeply, it requires a deeper reflexive recognition of the significance of technologies in articulating and maintaining the discursive ordering of social life. It also entails a posthumanist quest for the ontological conditions of selfhood, and in particular the renewal of practical reason as the primary mode of human agency, including the renewal of those moral traditions which articulate the deeper sources of our humanness.

This requires of us, therefore, a much greater critical reflexivity in relation to the dominant trajectory of technological innovation, and in particular to be able to recognise the ways in which technology expresses not just the political and commercial purposes of capitalism, but the instrumentalising and commodifying logic of instrumental reason. Choices about alternative technological trajectories and systems, about what sorts of regulatory regimes are in place to assess, monitor and redirect technologies are thus not only important expressions of a renewed active citizenship: they are also important sites for recovering the underlying political and ontological conditions of human selfhood and hence for the possibility of citizenship as a moral practice.

To conclude: I began this discussion by noting that, in the recent revival of interest in the language of citizenship, little attention has been given to the question of technology. I have argued that, rather than being seen as neutral tools, technologies need to be seen in more cultural and discursive terms, and that any meaningful recovery of the language and practice of citizenship will require a much greater technological reflexivity in general as well as the contestation of specific technologies within particular sites: domestic, workplace, R&D, public policy (Winner 1992). Whilst in this chapter I have tried to address the wider task of developing a more general reflexivity about technology, the other contributions to this volume address some of the particular sites in which the technological framing of active citizenship in a neo-liberal social context needs to be contested and negotiated.

Notes

1 I'm using the term 'active citizenship' here in a more general sense than that used in neo-liberal policy discourse, to encompass the various arguments for greater participation in civic life and the strengthening of public institutions.

2 However, analysts of neo-liberal governance are more interested in 'soft', social or 'meta' technologies, rather than specific areas of technological development, such as transportation, communication and the like (see Rose 1990).

3 See Winner's (1997) lament about the 'jarring irony' that, even though there is a consensus in the social studies of technology about the need for a constructivist approach to technology, public discourse on technology is dominated by instrumentalist and determinist views of technology.

4 For a discussion of the role of instrumental rationality in modern medicine, see Redding (1995).

5 See the discussion of the centrality of 'practice' in the special issue of *Inquiry* based on the paper by Charles Spinosa, Fernando Flores and Hubert L. Dreyfus (1995).

References

Aglietta, M. (1987) *A Theory of Capitalist Regulation: The US Experience*, trans. [from the French] David Fernbach, London: Verso.

Amin, A. (ed.) (1994) *Post-Fordism: A Reader*, Cambridge, MA: Blackwell.

Aronowitz, S., Martinsons, B. and Menser, M. (eds) (1996) *Technoscience and Cyberculture*, New York: Routledge.

Bauman, Z. (1992) *Intimations of Postmodernity*, London: Routledge.

Bauman, Z. (1997) *Postmodernity and its Discontents*, New York: New York University Press.

Beck, U. (1992) *Risk Society: Towards a New Modernity*, London: Sage.

Bijker, W.E., Hughes, T.P. and Pinch, T. (eds) (1987) *The Social Construction of Technological Systems: New Directions in the Sociology and History of Technology*, Cambridge, MA: MIT Press.

Borgmann, A. (1984) *Technology and the Character of Contemporary Life: A Philosophical Inquiry*, Chicago: University of Chicago Press.

Borgmann, A. (1992) *Crossing the Postmodern Divide*, Chicago: University of Chicago Press.

Burchell, D. (1995) 'The attributes of citizens: virtue, manners and the activity of citizenship', *Economy and Society*, 24, 4: 540–8.

Castells, M. (1997)*The Information Age: Economy, Society and Culture*, vol. II: *The Power of Identity*, Oxford: Basil Blackwell.

Clarke, S. (1990) 'The crisis of Fordism or the crisis of social democracy?' *Telos*, 83 (Spring): 71–98.

Cockburn, C. (1992) 'The circuit of technology: gender, identity and power', in R. Silverstone and E. Hirsch (eds), *Consuming Technologies: Media and Information in Domestic Spaces*, London: Routledge.

Cockburn, C. and Furst-Dilic, R. (eds) (1994) *Bringing Technology Home: Gender and Technology in a Changing Europe*, Milton Keynes: Open University Press.

Dosi, G. (1982) 'Technological paradigms and technological trajectories', *Research Policy*, 11: 147–62.

Drengson, A. (1995) *The Practice of Technology*, Albany, NY: SUNY.

Ellul, J. (1964) *The Technological Society*, New York: Vintage Books.

Emberley, P. (1989) 'Places and stories: the challenge of technology', *Social Research*, 56, 3: 744–5.

Fay, B. (1987) 'An alternative view: interpretive social science', in M.T. Gibbons (ed.), *Interpreting Politics*, Oxford: Basil Blackwell.

Featherstone, M. and Burrows, R. (1995) *Cyberspace, Cyberbodies, Cyberpunk: Culture of Technological Embodiment,* London: Sage.

Feenberg, A. (1992) 'Subversive rationalisation: technology, power and democracy', *Inquiry*, 35: 147–62.

Fieldes, D. and Bramble, T. (1992) 'Post-Fordism: historical break or utopian fantasy?', *Journal of Industrial Relations*, December: 562–79.

Foster, T. (1996) 'The sex appeal of the inorganic', in Robert Newman (ed.), *Centuries Ends, Narrative Means*, Stanford, CA: Stanford University Press.

Foucault, M. (1988) *Technologies of the Self: A Seminar with Michel Foucault,* (ed.) Luther H. Martin, Huck Gutman and Patrick H. Hutton, Amherst, MA : University of Massachusetts Press.

Gergen, K. (1991) *The Saturated Self: Dilemmas of Identity in Contemporary Life*, New York: Basic Books.

Giddens, A. (1991) *Modernity and Self Identity: Self and Society in the Late Modern Age*, Stanford, CA: Stanford University Press.

Grodin, D. and Lindlof, T. (1996) 'The self and mediated communication', in D. Grodin and T. Lindlof (eds), *Constructing the Self in a Mediated World*, Thousand Oaks, CA: Sage Publications.

Halberstam, J. and Livingston, I. (eds), (1995) *Posthuman Bodies*, Bloomington, IN: Indiana University Press.

Haraway, D. (1987) 'A manifesto for cyborgs: science, technology and socialist feminism in the 1980s', *Australian Feminist Studies* 4 (Autumn): 1–42.

Haraway, D. (1991a) Interview with Constance Penley and Andrew Ross, in C. Penley and A. Ross, (eds), *Technoculture*, Minneapolis: University of Minnesota Press.

Haraway, D. (1991b) *Simians, Cyborgs and Women: The Re-invention of Nature*, New York: Routledge.

Harvey, D. (1989) *The Condition of Postmodernity: An Enquiry into the Origins of Cultural Change*, Oxford: Basil Blackwell.

Heidegger, M. (1977) *The Question Concerning Technology, and Other Essays*, New York: Harper and Row.

Hill, S. (1988) *The Tragedy of Technology: Human Liberation vs Domination in the Late Twentieth Century*, London: Pluto Press.

Hinkson, J. (1993) 'Postmodern economy: self-formation, value and intellectual practice', *Arena Journal*, 1: 23–44.

Hirst, P. and Thompson, G. (1996) *Globalization in Question*, London: Polity Press.

Hirst, P. and Zeitlin, J. (1991) 'Flexible specialisation versus post-Fordism: theory, evidence and policy implications', *Economy and Society*, 20,1: 1–27.

Jameson, F. (1991) *Postmodernism of the Cultural Logic of Late Capitalism*, London: Verso.

Jessop, B. (1990) 'Regulation theories in retrospect and prospect', *Economy and Society*, 19, 2: 153–216.

Joerges, B. (1988) 'Technology in everyday life: conceptual queries', *Journal for the Theory of Social Behaviour*, 18, 2: 219–37.

Knight, J. (1995) 'Fading poststructuralisms: post-Ford, posthuman, post-education?', in R. Smith and P. Wexler (eds), *After Post-modernism: Education, Politics and Identity*, London: Falmer Press.

Kroker, A. (1992) *The Possessed Individual: Technology and the French Postmodern*, New York: St Martin's Press.

Lash, S. and Urry, J. (1994) *Economies of Signs and Space*, London: Sage.

Loader, B. (ed.) (1997) *The Governance of Cyberspace: Politics, Technology and Global Restructuring*, London: Routledge.

Lodge, D. (1989) *Nice Work*, Harmondsworth, Middx: Penguin Books.

Mathews, J. (1989) *Age of Democracy: The Politics of Post-Fordism*, Melbourne: Oxford University Press.

Meredyth, D. (1997) 'Invoking citizenship: education, competence and social rights', *Economy and Society*, 26, 2: 273–295.

Misa, T. (1988) 'How machines make history, and how historians (and others) help them to do so', *Science, Technology and Human Values*, 13, 3 and 4: 308–31.

Morgan, M. (1994) 'Religion, history and moral discourse', in J.Tully (ed.), *Philosophy in an Age of Pluralism: The Philosophy of Charles Taylor in Question*, Cambridge: Cambridge University Press.

Morley, D. and Silverstone, R. (1990) 'Domestic communication: technologies and meanings', *Media, Culture and Society*, 12: 31–55.

Mouffe, C. (1988) 'The civics lesson', *New Statesman and Society*, October: 1–18, 28–30.

Muetzelfeldt, M. (1992) 'Economic rationalism in its social context', in M. Muetzelfeldt (ed.), *Society, State and Politics in Australia*, Sydney, NSW: Pluto Press.

Noble, D. (1977) *America by Design: Science, Technology and the Rise of Corporate Capitalism*, New York: A.E. Knopf.

Penley, C. and Ross, A. (eds), (1991) *Technoculture*, Minneapolis: University of Minnesota Press.

Perez, C. (1983) 'Structural change and assimilation of new technologies in the economic and social systems', *Futures*, October: 357–75.

Pippin, R. (1995) 'On the notion of technology as ideology', in A. Feenberg and A. Hannay (eds), *Technology and the Politics of Knowledge*, Bloomington, IN: Indiana University Press.

Poster, M. (1994) 'A second media age?', *Arena Journal*, 3: 49–89.

Redding, P. (1995) 'Science, medicine and illness: rediscovering the patient as a person', in P.A. Komesaroff (ed.), *Troubled Bodies: Critical Perspectives on Postmodernism, Medical Ethics and the Body*, Carlton: Melbourne University Press.

Roobeek, A.J. (1987) 'The crisis in Fordism and the rise of a new technological paradigm', *Futures*, April: 129–54.

Rose, N. (1990) 'Obliged to be free', in *Governing the Soul: Technologies of Human Subjectivity*, London: Routledge.

Sclove, R. (1995) *Democracy and Technology*, New York: Guilford Press.

Scrinis, G. (1997) 'Road to nowhere', *The Age*, 24 January: A15.

Silverstone, R. (1989) 'Let us return to the murmuring of everyday prac-tices: a note on Michel de Certeau, television and everyday life', *Theory, Culture and Society*, 6: 77–94.

Silverstone, R. and Hirsch, E. (eds) (1992) *Consuming Technologies: Media and Information in Domestic Spaces*, London: Routledge.

Skinner, Q. (1994) 'Modernity and disenchantment: some historical reflections', in J. Tully (ed.), *Philosophy in an Age of Pluralism: The Philosophy of Charles Taylor in Question*, Cambridge: Cambridge University Press.

Sobchak, V. (1995) 'Beating the meat/surviving the text, or how to get out of this century alive' in M. Featherstone and R. Burrows (eds), *Cyberspace, Cyberbodies, Cyberpunk: Culture of Technological Embodiment*, London: Sage.

Spinosa, C., Flores, F. and Dreyfus, H.L.. (1995) 'Disclosing new worlds: entrepreneurship, democratic action, and the cultivation of solidarity', *Inquiry*, 38, 1–2: 3–64.

Taylor, C. (1989) *Sources of the Self: The Making of the Modern Identity*, Cambridge, MA: Harvard University Press.

Taylor, C. (1993) 'Engaged agency and background in Heidegger', in C. Guignon (ed.), *A Cambridge Companion to Heidegger*, Cambridge: Cambridge University Press.

Thiele, L.P. (1995) 'Receiving the sky and awaiting divinities', in L.P. Thiele, *Timely Meditations: Martin Heidegger and Postmodern Politics*, Princeton, NJ: Princeton University Press.

Turkle, S. (1984) *The Second Self: The Human Spirit in a Computer Culture*, New York: Simon and Schuster.

Turkle, S. (1995) *Life on the Screen: Identity in the Age of the Internet*, New York: Simon and Schuster.

Winner, L. (1986a) 'Do artefacts have politics?', in L. Winner, *The Whale and the Reactor: A Search for Limits in an Age of High Technology*, Chicago: University of Chicago Press.

Winner, L. (1986b) 'Technologies as forms of life', in *The Whale and the Reactor: A Search for Limits in an Age of High Technology*, Chicago: University of Chicago Press.

Winner, L. (1992) 'Citizen virtues in a technological order', *Inquiry*, 35: 341–61.

Winner, L. (1997) 'Technology today: Utopia or dystopia?', in 'Technology and the Rest of Culture', special issue of *Social Research*, 64, 3: 990–1017.

Wynne, B. (1988) 'Unruly technology: practical rules, impractical discourses and public understanding', *Social Studies of Science*, 18: 146–67.

Zimmerman, M. (1990) *Heidegger's Confrontation with Modernity: Technology, Politics, Art*, Bloomington, IN: Indiana University Press.

Zuboff, S. (1988) *In the Age of the Smart Machine*, New York: Basic Books.

Question from Alan: One of your criticisms of policy conceptions of technology is of the failure to acknowledge the constitutive importance of technologies; the ways in which they are implicated in ongoing processes of self-constitution. I think your criticism is a valid and important one. However, I was wondering how this fits with your argument, outlined later in the chapter, about the need to 'recover' the 'ontological conditions of selfhood'. This seems to reinstate the notion of the authentic self. Aren't the conditions of selfhood themselves at least in part reconfigured by technology?

Response: Before I try to answer the two basic parts of your question: whether I'm seeking to reinstate the notion of an authentic self and whether the conditions of selfhood are themselves altered by technology, I'd like to develop a bit more why I think that talking about recovering the ontological conditions of selfhood is an important and legitimate part of our project.

It seems to me that a poststructuralist account of the rationalities of rule is very powerful in its deconstruction of the language of liberal practices: freedom, autonomy, responsibility, rights, citizenship and so on, as part of the apparatus of liberal governance. Yet in so doing it raises the question of whether it does so without remainder. For this language is central to the sense of self-identity, personal relationships and political agency that structures our own everyday lived experience of the world. To deconstruct such language in terms of the operation of fields of power opens up the question: Is that all there is? Of course, as academics we can try to bracket that question as outside our scholarly brief. However, in our own embodied, everyday experience, which includes the academic practices of reading, writing and teaching about the expressions of power/knowledge, we do not stand above the processes we are talking about. What do we make of our own agency and self-identity, and of the language of rights, dignity, autonomy, responsibility, care and so on?

In my view, then, a necessary practical corollary of deconstructing rationalities of rule is the task of reflection, within our everyday social practices, of the ontological conditions of that sense of self and relationality which is integral to those practices. Not to do so means perhaps that we ourselves become, by default, part of the technologies of liberal governance.

For example, in the academic practices we share in common, what do we make of the ongoing reconstruction of the university in terms of the language and ethos of neo-liberalism? Presumably we continue to regard our students as persons with rights, dignity, feelings and dreams, for whom undergraduate and postgraduate studies are not simply means to a good job and a steady income, but participation in communal scholarly traditions which embody a sense of what it means to be human. Yet we are aware of the ways in which the new managerialism does affect the ways in which we think about students, and more generally what we regard as acceptable, indeed 'thinkable', academic practice. Early in 1998, the Vice-Chancellor and Pro-Vice-Chancellor of Research of Melbourne University pressured the Board of Melbourne University Press to reject a manuscript edited by Tony Coady from the University's Philosophy Department which examined the idea of the university from a viewpoint critical of the trend towards corporatism. The reason? Because it was insufficiently balanced. Censorship of scholarship by corporate managers because such scholarship is mildly critical of a university's corporate image has, it seems, become acceptable university practice.

In this context I'm reminded of a gloomy comment made by Stuart Hall in 1993 in response to the Thatcherite reforms of British higher education:

> One of the key lessons I learned from Thatcherism was that first of all you struggle about conduct, and hearts and minds follow later. I learnt that through the institution in which I work, the Open University. It is filled with good social democrats. Everybody there believes in the redistribution of educational opportunities and seeks to remedy the exclusiveness of British education. And yet, in the past ten years, these good social democratic souls, without changing for a minute what is in their hearts and minds, have learned to speak a brand of metallic entrepreneurialism, a new managerialism of a horrendously closed nature. They believe what they always believed, but what they do, how they write their mission statements, how they do their appraisal forms, how they talk about their students, how they calculate the cost – that's what they are really interested in now. The result is that the institution has been transformed.
>
> (Hall 1993: 15)

The lesson I draw from this is that, in so far as we are opposed to the managerialist transformation of the university, we need not only to maintain those practices of teaching, research and administration which embody a sense of normative purpose but also to articulate an alternative language of moral and political resistance.

In your question you suggest that I want to reinstate the notion of an authentic self. I presume by that you mean some idea of an 'essential' or presocial self. That's not what I'm proposing. I'm not talking about some kind of pre-social essence, a punctual self which precedes the linguistic practices of selfhood. As I indicated in my chapter, what I am arguing for is something along the lines of Charles Taylor's account of the self in *Sources of the Self* (Taylor 1989). Taylor's account of the self is not an essentialist one and, like poststructuralism, he recognises that the self is constituted in and through social processes. Indeed, in *Sources of the Self*, Taylor develops a genealogical account of those moral sources which still sustain (though in considerably modified form) what he calls the modern identity. Central to Taylor's account is his assertion that to be a self is to be necessarily orientated in moral space, a space of questions, embodied answers to which constitute us as selves. Taylor insists that such 'moral frameworks' are not optional extras, which we could choose to live without if we wanted to, but are integral to being human. They only seem optional because of the distorting influence of modern epistemology and reductive theories of human life. Against such reductivism Taylor's task has been to recover the importance of moral ontology, though not through an objectivist epistemology, but through the recovery of the language of lived practical rationality or what he calls 'moral phenom- enology'. It might be worth quoting Taylor's own summary account of this:

> What I first described as 'frameworks' I presented as offering back- ground assumptions to our moral reactions, and later as providing the contexts in which these reactions have sense. Then I went on to argue that living in these frameworks was not an optional extra, something we might just as well do without, but that they provided a kind of orientation essential to our identity. What seemed to make it necessary to say all this was the resistance put up by the natural- istic temper which pervades all our philosophical thought, not only within the academy but in our society at large. The mode of thought which surfaces in contemporary sociobiology wants us to think of our moral reactions outside of any sense-making context, as on all fours with visceral reactions like nausea. On a more sophisticated

level, we have the picture of values as projections on a neutral world, something which we normally live within but could perhaps abstain from. It has been necessary to describe all this at length in order to rescue our awareness of the crucial importance of these distinctions [i.e. what Taylor calls 'qualitative discriminations' of basic goods through which articulate our moral orientation] from a kind of bewitchment.

(Taylor 1989: 10).

Second, with respect to whether technologies alter the conditions of selfhood. I agree that they do. My argument is that when taken in their full depth and complexity, modern technologies alter our social practices in ways that shape our subjectivities and social identities within a framework of instrumental rationality which disconnects us from the moral sources Taylor is talking about. I believe that to flourish as selves in a technological context thus requires languages and practices which resist the processes of instrumentalisation, commodification and disenchantment and sustain some kind of moral orientation.

Albert Borgmann, who, like Taylor, has drawn on Heidegger's critique of technological enframement, talks about the need for what he calls 'focal practices' through which we articulate personal and communal self-identity in and through a practical engagement with material life. Borgmann recognises that technologies, far from being external to the processes of self-formation, are integral to becoming and being a self. His contribution has been to take seriously the seemingly trivial meanings of technologies within everyday practices and to argue for a more critical, normative re-engagement with the real, something which he calls 'postmodern realism' in *Crossing the Postmodern Divide* (Borgmann 1992).

One of the problems with Borgmann's approach in his earlier book, *Technology and the Character of Contemporary Life* (1984) was that it gave the impression, at least, that in order to resist the commodifying effects of the 'device paradigm' we needed to recover more or less 'pretechnological' practices such as the experience of wilderness. The problem with this, as with forms of radical environmentalism, is that it uncritically assumes a nature–culture division, although one in which a supposedly unmediated access to 'nature' provides us with a basic moral orientation (Soper 1995). It is also of little practical help in making moral sense of urban technological practices. In *Crossing the Postmodern Divide* Borgmann gives more attention to how we might recover 'focal practices' within the context of urbanised, media-saturated and technologically intensive life worlds. In particular, he alerts us to the need to recognise and to contest the ways in which 'hypermodern' technologies transform us as persons and communities.

This process of subtle transformation through the technological modification of our social practices is evident in the changing meanings of the languages of community, communication, freedom, rights and so on. As many people have observed, these words become redefined instrumentally, in terms of the technologies themselves, thus extending the inversion of means and ends. Thus communication as a primary human need or right becomes redefined in terms of access to communication technologies. It is in fact the process of the 'colonisation of the life world' described by Habermas (1984: 342) and needs to be resisted, not just by maintaining procedural rights and equalities, but by opening up questions of social ontology: what kinds of people are we or are we becoming?

References

Borgmann, A. (1984) *Technology and the Character of Contemporary Life: A Philosophical Inquiry*, Chicago: University of Chicago Press.

Borgmann, A. (1992) *Crossing the Postmodern Divide*, Chicago: University of Chicago Press.

Habermas, J. (1984) *Theory of Communicative Action*, vol. 1, trans. T. McCarthy, Boston, MA: Beacon Press.

Hall, S. (1993) 'Thatcherism today', *New Statesman and Society*, 26, November: 15.

Soper, K. (1995) 'Feminism and ecology: realism and rhetoric in the discourses of nature', *Science, Technology and Human Values*, 20, 3: 311 –31.

Taylor, C. (1989) *Sources of the Self: The Making of the Modern Identity*, Cambridge: Cambridge University Press.

Question from Patricia: Your chapter is a critique of instrumental reason – as mediated by the practices of technology – and you are calling for a re-engagement with the moral dimensions of the self and with the practice of citizenship. Further, you refer to citizenship variously as a moral practice, as moral agency and as engaged agency. I'd be interested in your clarifying your conception of citizenship, or discussing it further. If you are talking of citizenship in terms of the civic republican tradition, how do you accommodate this ontological notion with the critiques of 'community' and ontological citizenship by such writers as Iris Marion Young?

Response: Yes, in talking about citizenship in terms a moral practice I am drawing to some extent on contemporary civic republican ideas. However, of course I recognise that it is neither possible nor desirable to apply an 'ideal type' civic republican model to the circumstances of a contemporary liberal democratic polity. I also agree with David Burchell (1995) that much of the debate over civic republicanism suffers from a romanticism which mystifies the citizen as a transcendental subject. Yet whilst Burchell is right to emphasise the ways in which 'citizens' are formed in and through the external activities of government and the internal practices of self-discipline, this still leaves open the significance of citizenship as a normative oppositional discourse in the context of the neo-liberal reconstruction of public life. I agree with Chantall Mouffe's (1988) argument that civic republicanism provides a valuable resource for a radical democratic critique of the practices, discourses and institutions of neo-liberalism, particularly with respect to conceptions of political agency, the divisions between public and private spheres, and the relationship between individual rights and common goods. Put simply, as our practices and identities are pervasively reconstituted in terms of consumption, the language of citizenship has the potential to articulate an alternative.

Like Bowles and Gintis (1986), I believe that the task of radical democracy is to extend and enrich rather than to displace liberal and socialist practices and discourses of rights, citizenship and community. As Mouffe (1988: 30) commented in the context of Tory attempts to appropriate the language of 'active citizenship' at the end of the Thatcher era in Britain:

> One thing is certain. A purely defensive strategy to reassert the liberal view of the citizen as a bearer of rights is inadequate. It may help us resist the neo-liberal onslaught on existing rights, but it is not enough. To be able to formulate a satisfactory notion of the political community we must go beyond liberal individualism to questions of justice, equality and community as well.

In trying to answer the two parts of your question I shall first expand a little more on the ways in which a civic republican perspective can modify liberal practices and discourses. Then I shall consider Iris Marion

Young's (1989, 1996) argument that the universalist notion of citizenship and the emphasis on 'the common good' characteristic of the civic republican traditions and argument do not allow the recognition of 'the positivity of group difference'. It is my view that certain features of republicanism, particularly the idea of a 'thicker' public sphere, the renegotiation of the relationship between public and private spheres, and an orientation towards public argument about shared or common goods can actually be more conducive to the expression of group difference than her proposals for a more heterogeneous public sphere or for the idea of a communicative democracy.

From a radical democratic perspective (and situated within the pervasive practices and institutions of a neo-liberal social order) civic republicanism contributes a number of key ideas for the critique and reconstruction of liberalism. One is a richer conception of public life, as a space not just for the pursuit of preformed interests governed by procedural rules, but for human flourishing and for civic argument and deliberation about substantive issues. A second is a conception of citizenship as a practice, and not just a legal status with associated rights. As Skinner (1992) suggests, a modern republican conception of political agency may in fact provide a surer ground for the protection of rights, and certainly for resistance against their continuing refashioning as forms of regulation. In republican terms, it is also a reflexive and constitutive practice, involving political learning and the formation of individual identity and collective identity through political deliberation (Marquand 1988, 1997; Jordan 1989). A liberal view of political activity tends to be more instrumentalist, such that politics becomes the negotiation between preformed interests, with little prospect for change and learning (Young 1996).

A third is the notion of common purposes which are larger than a collection of private preferences (Jordan 1989). Before we talk about the dangers of a hegemonic common good we should recognise what the distinction between a civic and a consumerist orientation means in practical terms, for example in our attitudes to environmental conservation and the use of resources. The practices of recycling, of more ecologically responsible use of public transport, and also of buying locally made goods express a civic sense of belonging to a community with shared interests which may at times conflict with our immediate consumer preferences.

I want to turn now to the second part of your question, which has to do with Iris Marion Young's claim that a civic republican conception of public life, no less than that of modern liberalism, suppresses difference:

> The ideal of a civic public, I have argued, excludes women and other groups as different, because its rational and universal status derives only from its opposition to affectivity, particularity, and the body. Republican theorists insisted on the unity of the civic public: insofar as he is a citizen every man leaves behind his particularity and difference, to adopt a universalist standpoint identical for all citizens, the standpoint of the common good or the general will.
>
> (Young 1989: 117)

Young (ibid.: 166) argues against any notion of citizenship based upon an idea of commonality or common good which transcends group differences. Indeed, she argues for the assertion of the positivity of group difference over against the pluralism of liberalism humanism:

> a politics that asserts the positivity of group difference is liberating and empowering. In the act of reclaiming the identity the dominant culture has taught them to despise . . . , and affirming it as an identity to celebrate, the oppressed remove double consciousness. I am just what they say I am – a Jewboy, a colored girl, a fag, a dyke, or a hag – and proud of it. No longer does one have the impossible project of trying to become something one is not under circumstances where the very trying reminds one of who one is. This politics asserts that oppressed groups have distinct cultures, experiences, and perspectives on social life with humanly positive meaning, some of which may even be superior to the culture and perspectives of mainstream society. The rejection and devaluation of one's culture and perspective should not be a condition of full participation in social life.

This statement contains a number of objections to the republican tradition: first, that it devalues the affectivity and particularity of the body by relegating it to the private sphere; and second, that the idea of a common good suppresses difference. In opposition to this, Young argues for a more heterogeneous public sphere which rejects notions of common good and an inclusive 'public'.

In her more recent essay, 'Communication and the other: beyond deliberative democracy', Young (1996) argues for a communicative democracy which enables a more effective expression of difference. She expresses her partial agreement with theorists of deliberative democracy against an interest based model of democracy. However, she reiterates her opposition to any notion of ontological unity:

> The unity of a single polity is a much weaker unity, I suggest, than deliberative theorists usually assume. The unity that motivates politics is the facticity of people being thrown together, finding themselves in geographical proximity and economic interdependence such that activities and pursuits of some affect the ability of others to conduct their activities. A polity consists of people who live together, who are stuck with one another ... If a polity is to be a communicative democracy ... its members must have a commitment to equal respect for one another, in the simple formal sense of willingness to say that all have a right to express their opinions and points of view and all ought to listen. The members of the polity, furthermore, must agree on procedural rules of fair discussion and decision making. These three conditions − significant interdependence, formally equal respect, and agreed on procedures − are all the unity necessary for communicative democracy. They are much thinner conditions than those of shared understanding or the goals of finding common goods.
>
> (Young 1996: 126)

In brief, my argument is this: yes, I support the development of a more heterogeneous public life, where there is greater expression of difference. However, I believe that the resources of the republican tradition better enable us to foster such expression of difference than Young allows. Further, I think that Young is insufficiently reflexive with respect to the universalism of her own taken-for-granted enlightenment framework. Her position is close to a cosmopolitan liberalism which has difficulty in genuinely recognising the more substantive differences between alternative forms of life, and tends to reduce difference to matters of lifestyle choice and consumer preference. In other words, I think that the 'positivity of group difference' entails going much further than she does. I suggest that it requires a more thoroughgoing recognition of the deeper incommensurability of alternative forms of life and also of the ways in which enlightenment liberalism, particularly in its late modern form of a globalising technocapitalism, itself constitutes an overarching form of life.

A failure to engage in this more thoroughgoing dialogical reflection involves either a 'tolerance' which is a tacit negation of the other as less civilised, or a tacit assimilation, such that 'difference' is modified in such a way that it is presumed to be within the meta-frame of enlightenment assumptions.

With respect to the first, Zygmunt Bauman (1992: xxiii–xxiv) has commented:

> A truly consistent rejection of the heteronomy entailed in the monologic stance would lead, paradoxically, to lofty and derisive indifference. One would need, after all, to refrain from prompting the other to act according to the rules one accepts as morally sound, and from preventing the other following rules one views as odious and abominable; such self-restraint, however, cannot be easily detached from its corollary: the disdainful view of the other as an essentially inferior being, one that need not or cannot lift himself or be lifted to the level of life viewed as properly human. One may say that the zealous avoidance of the monologic stance leads to consequences strikingly similar to those one wished to stave off. If I consider corporal punishment degrading and bodily mutations inhuman, letting the others to practice them in the name of the right to choose (or because I cannot believe any more in the universality of moral rules) amounts to the re-assertion of my own superiority: 'they may wallow in barbarities I would never put up with ... that serves them right, those savages'. The renunciation of the monologic stance does not seem, therefore an unmixed blessing. The more radical it is, the more it resembles moral relativism in its behavioural incarnation of callous indifference.

The other unsatisfactory response is tacitly to assimilate difference within the taken-for-granted meta-narrative of a universalising modernity. As Fullinwinder (1996: 40) comments:

> 'Pluralism', then, contains unspoken qualifications – about what is really worth respecting, affirming, or valuing in a culture, whether our own or others. Its grounding postulate of mutual respect may require substantial cultural changes – in short a good deal of as-similation – by some groups. Establishing a multicultural society based on mutual respect may require groups to revise their attitudes towards law and law-abidingness; education and open-mindedness;

race gender and intermarriage; public expression of opinions and interests; and religious toleration. It surely requires induction of all members into a common core culture, since mutual respect does not live in isolation from specific cultural forms and supports.

Young's position, then, has I believe the same kinds of problems that Stanley Fish has identified with respect to what he calls 'boutique multiculturalism' (Fish 1997). Fish argues that even a 'strong multiculturalism' which celebrates diversity with respect to cultural life still tacitly assumes a larger framework of enlightenment modernity, such that eventually there are significant limits. There are boundaries beyond which difference may not go.

In an unreflective multicultural liberalism, such practices as infanticide, polygamy are seen to violate the very basis of civility, tolerance, expression of difference. I'm not saying that it is wrong to take such a view. What is wrong is to fail to recognise the universalist assumptions involved: that even as we celebrate the 'difference' of marginalised groups, we do so on the assumption that they can ultimately be contained within a common progressive, emancipatory vision of the world.

What is needed is an appreciation that the thoroughgoing recognition of the positivity of group difference entails an opening up not only of different practices, but also the conceptions of truth, goodness and beauty upon which these depend. Hence, a genuinely pluralistic society will engage in more fundamental debate about different forms of life and social visions, with the recognition that incommensurable forms of life entail different conceptions of truth, of justice and of community.

This applies of course to western liberalism as well: that, as Charles Taylor (1992) puts it, enlightenment liberalism is itself a fighting creed, construing the social world in its own particular way. What I am suggesting is that, paradoxically, genuine pluralism entails not the effective repression of universalistic claims, but rather the more explicit acknowledgment of such claims, and a clearer differentiation of the deeper agonistic disagreements between incommensurable forms of life.

A politics of difference which goes beyond a taken-for-granted enlightenment liberalism by articulating the implicit metanarratives of different forms of life could draw on the resources of a civic republicanism, particularly in terms of its non-instrumentalist conception of public life and its conception of 'the public' as an essentially contested space of self-constitution. It could also draw on the renegotiation of the differences between public and private life, such that those more fundamental and incommensurable disagreements which within a liberal conception tend to be relegated to the private sphere are given clearer recognition as constitutive of public life.

Drawing on these resources means, not the adoption of notions of 'the common good' in an ontological sense, but rather as provisional agreement with respect to limited political purposes. I'm suggesting therefore that the resources of a civic republican conception of politics as civic practice will help to reconceptualise (rather than dissolve) the public/private division in a way that protects the differences of minority groups by placing limits on any totalising 'common good'.

References

Bauman, Z. (1992) *Intimations of Postmodernity*, London: Routledge.

Bowles, S. and Gintis, H. (1986) *Democracy and Capitalism: Property, Community and the Contradictions of Modern Social Thought*, New York: Basic Books.

Burchell, D. (1995) 'The attributes of citizens: virtue, manners and the activity of citizenship', *Economy and Society*, 24, 4: 540–58.

Fish, S. (1997) 'Boutique multiculturalism, or why liberals are incapable of thinking about hate speech', *Critical Inquiry*, 23 (Winter): 378–418.

Fullinwinder, R. (1996) 'The cosmopolitan community', *Journal of Social Philosophy*, 27, 2: 32–50.

Jordan, B. (1989) *The Common Good: Citizenship, Morality and Self Interest*, Oxford: Basil Blackwell.

Marquand, D. (1988) *The Unprincipled Society: New Demands and Old Politics*, London: Jonathan Cape.

Marquand, D. (1997) *The New Reckoning: Capitalism, States and Citizens*, Cambridge: Polity Press.

Mouffe, C. (1988) 'The civics lesson', *New Statesman and Society*, October: 1–18, 28–30.

Skinner, Q. (1992) 'On justice, the common good and the priority of liberty', in C. Mouffe (ed.), *Dimensions of Radical Democracy: Pluralism, Citizenship, Community*, London: Verso.

Taylor, C. (1992) *Multiculturalism and 'the Politics of Recognition': An Essay*, ed. A. Gutmann, Princeton, NJ: Princeton University Press.

Young, I.M. (1989) 'Polity and group difference: a critique of the ideal of universal citizenship', *Ethics*, 99: 250–74.

Young, I.M. (1996) 'Communication and the other: beyond deliberative democracy', in Selya Benhabib (ed.), *Democracy and Difference: Contesting the Boundaries of the Political*, Princeton, NJ: Princeton University Press.

Question from Janice: Ian, you are critical of the instrumental nature of the technological triumphalism which characterises much of western society at the end of the twentieth century. You are arguing for the recovery of a more human centred citizenship through 'engaged agency', through 'practical reason' and through a 'world of involvement'.

Burchell, Rose and others working with the notion of governmentality analyse advanced liberal governance as government through the agency of the 'responsible' citizen. Can you clarify the ways in which you differentiate between these forms of agency? Is it that the advanced liberal governance described by Rose and others is directed towards particular outcomes, whereas you are privileging the practice of agency, with contingent outcomes resulting from negotiation?

Response: I think there are some points of agreement between the critiques of liberal agency (and hence 'citizenship') developed by governmentality theorists and what I will call 'civic humanists' (including civic republicans, communitarians, radical democrats and so on), but also deeper disagreements.

Governmentality theorists (GTs) and civic humanists (CHs) are in agreement that the neo-liberal rhetoric (and self-understanding) of increased freedom is inadequate or illusory. Neo-liberals of course imagine that what they are doing is recovering and enhancing individual freedom, choice, responsibility by rolling back the regulatory and coercive powers of the state. However, GTs and CHs differ significantly in terms of their 'deconstructive' accounts of neo-liberal agency. I'll talk about these in terms of the respective sociological analyses, epistemological critiques and prospects for normative alternatives they develop.

Social analysis: GTs analyse liberal ideas of freedom, autonomy, responsibility in terms of their functional importance for neo-liberal forms of governance: what you have described as 'steering at a distance'. In this account, rather than the exercise of individual freedom being antithetical to governmental regulation and control, it is actually central to a distinctively intensive rather than extensive regulation. I think that this mode of analysis is particularly illuminating of a range of policy developments and practices, such as the areas of social policy, higher education and genetic medicine, which you and the others have discussed.

By contrast, the CHs interpret neo-liberal forms of agency as corrosive of the social conditions and civic virtues needed to maintain genuine civic freedom and ensure the efficient functioning of a limited and responsive state. A good example of this CH approach is Christopher Lasch's critique of liberal modernity in *The Culture of Narcissism* (1979) and *The Minimal Self* (1984). In Lasch's view the decline of the informal networks of neighbourhood life and hence local knowledges and traditions associated with the increasing atomisation and commodification of everyday life has led to a corresponding expansion in the role of bureaucrats, experts, various kinds of propagandists and law enforcement agencies. Hence, liberal freedom is increasingly illusory.

It is interesting that these different critiques of neo-liberal conceptions of increasing individual freedoms suggest quite different scenarios for the further diffusion of neo-liberal forms of governance. A governmentalisation analysis suggests, perhaps, ever more sophisticated forms of 'self-regulation' and self-monitoring, whilst a CH analysis suggests the increasing ungovernability of a neo-liberal social order resulting from the depletion of 'social capital' or the erosion of civil society institutions.

Epistemological critique: These different interpretations of a neo-liberal social order reflect quite different epistemological critiques of the more or less instrumentalist or representationalist views of truth of liberal modernity. GTs of course reject a modernist representational epistemology, arguing instead for the discursive construction of social life and agency within regimes of truth.

Whilst it is hard to generalise, CHs tend to talk in terms of the critique of instrumental rationality and the recovery of 'practical reason'. A good example of this is Alasdair Macintyre's *After Virtue* (1984). In brief, MacIntyre argues that the enlightenment project of articulating a universalist rational morality (i.e. Kantian deontology and utilitarianism) within the epistemological framework of instrumental reason has failed, with the result that the language of morality has collapsed into emotivism in which there is no clear distinction between manipulative and non-manipulative social relations. That is to say, within the Weberian separation of means and ends, facts and values, it has not been possible to articulate universally agreed moral principles. Although we still use the language of values and ends, this language has become increasingly fragmented and incoherent, and regarded as merely subjective preferences. Furthermore, social discourse becomes increasingly instrumental in character, a claim which MacIntyre illustrates by referring to what he describes as the paradigmatic characters of late modern social life: the aesthete, the therapist, the manager and the bureaucratic expert.

Prospects for recovery: Thus, I think that both GTs and CHs are describing the consequences of the dominance of an instrumental rationality for liberal humanist conceptions of moral agency, especially within the microstructures of everyday life. Both draw our attention to the ways in which subjectivities are shaped by and are in turn expressive of the instrumental rationality of 'the market' and the neo-liberal bureaucracy. What I find most disconcerting is the 'instrumentalisation' of the whole range of human relationships, where the languages of care, responsiveness, flexibility and so on become essentially manipulative 'technologies'.

However, where they differ is in relation to the possibility of any epistemological alternative to dominant (instrumentalist) 'rationalities of rule'. As I understand it, GTs don't wish to theorise alternatives to regimes of truth in epistemological terms. Their more 'modest' task is to deconstruct them and stir some forms of resistance. By contrast, CHs like MacIntyre argue for a return to older Aristotelian traditions of practical reason, civic virtue and the like. MacIntyre's general argument is that, rather than the kind of abstract universalist theories of utilitarian and Kantian liberalism, we need to recover an understanding of morality which is grounded in a teleological account of the development of human character and virtue, which is undergirded by a communal narrative and expressed through specific social practices.

MacIntyre has been criticised as being unremittingly anti-modern and not much help in terms of how we are supposed to recover practical reason in the context of technological modernity (including those social practices through which we acquire those virtues that make it possible for us to act freely as socially embedded persons). I guess that it is to this kind of challenge that I was in part alluding in my essay.

References

Lasch, C. (1979) *The Culture of Narcissism: American Life in an Age of Diminishing Expectations*, New York: W.W. Norton.

Lasch, C. (1984) *The Minimal Self: Psychic Survival in Troubled Times*, New York: W.W. Norton.

MacIntyre, A. (1984) *After Virtue: A Study in Moral Theory*, Notre Dame, IN: University of Notre Dame Press.

Chapter 6

Conclusion

Ian Barns, Janice Dudley, Patricia Harris and Alan Petersen

At the very beginning of this book we discussed the need for policy makers and policy analysts who are concerned about protecting and advancing rights to appraise basic concepts and categories critically in the light of the emergence of economic liberalism, the reconstruction of the welfare state and so on. Poststructuralism, we argued, offers a unique kind of deconstructive and analytic approach that profoundly challenges the ways in which we understand the human, and the terms by which we describe and analyse social policy. Poststructuralists challenge the notion that there is an overall pattern in history and that the present state of affairs is inevitable and immutable. Governmentality scholars, in particular, have sought to expose the operations and diverse manifestations of an increasingly dominant form of rule known as advanced liberalism or neo-liberalism, thereby allowing us to imagine that things could be otherwise. In different ways each chapter has attempted to make visible the rationality of rule of neo-liberalism and the ways in which populations in advanced capitalist societies are governed through a regime of increasingly contractual relations between people. One of the major purposes in doing this has been to open up spaces for contestation and for the emergence of alternative social rationalities.

One of the central concepts with which we have been concerned in this book is that of 'citizenship'. In the respective sites of welfare provision, higher education, the emerging genetic-based public health and the diffusion of new technologies in everyday life, we have attempted to demonstrate the ambiguous and essentially contested meanings of citizenship, and in particular the ways in which citizenship has been articulated in terms of the active entrepreneurial subject of neo-liberal governance. At the same time we have also raised the possibilities of citizenship as an alternative language of resistance and the defence of the social. Patricia Harris spoke of the contestation of the marketisation of welfare which appealed to wider values: democratic rights, participation, economic equality and social stability. Janice Dudley spoke of policies of citizenship education which might counter current policies which privilege neo-classical economics and neo-liberal politics: citizenship education could engage with difference and could articulate ideals such as cultural pluralism, indigenous reconciliation and inclusivity. Alan Petersen focused on the potential of lay knowledges, or the 'rationalities employed by lay people in decision making in relation to the new genetics', in making genetics an important site for contesting the meanings of citizenship. Finally, Ian Barns spoke of the ways in which citizenship requires a reflexive recognition of the constitutive significance of new technologies and the creation of new forms of public deliberation about technological possibilities.

In this final chapter we raise the question of how the more critical understanding of citizenship might be useful to people involved in the policy process, as policy makers, policy activists or as citizens. It is based on an edited transcript of an audio-taped discussion among Alan, Ian, Janice and Patricia which explores the ways in which the language of 'citizenship' can be developed as a language of resistance and/or of governance in each of our four areas.

Specifically, we discussed whether we thought 'citizenship' could be deployed as a language of resistance to neo-liberalism and articulated as an alternative 'rationality of rule' that might help to recover the social. We also debated the specific practices which an alternative conception of citizenship might entail (for example, in welfare provision, higher education, genetic-based public health, technology practices and so on).

Citizenship as language

IAN: Can 'citizenship' be used as a language of resistance against neo-liberalism and its policies and practices, or does it tend to become coopted and thus just a component of neo-liberal rationalities of rule?

PATRICIA: Both, because there is not one language of citizenship. There are multiple languages of citizenship. Citizenship talk as used by neo-liberals is problematic for all the reasons we have pointed out in the chapters.

IAN: Isn't the problem of neo-liberalism that it coopts the term citizenship and locates it within a market discourse so that the metanarrative is one of the competitive market?

ALAN: An assumption underlying our discussion is that citizenship has been hijacked by the New Right or the neo-liberals. But the recent emergence of discussion about citizenship ... [is] in large part due to the agitations of new social movements, for example the new feminist, civil rights movements and ecological movement ... gay rights, etc. So once you start phrasing the argument in terms of neo-liberal imperatives then in a way you are accepting that it's holding the floor. But as we started off by saying, there are many discourses of citizenship ...

JANICE: Citizenship is about membership of an imagined community, and the rights and entitlements that come from that membership. And, certainly in the twentieth century, it has been inextricably linked to the notion of the nation-state. So, in democratic states, there is this blurring between notions of citizenship rights and notions of human rights, and for a whole variety of reasons, not the least of which is countries being signatories to international agreements, ... there is a degree of congruence between citizenship rights and human rights in democratic states. I think we'd agree that we are talking about citizenship in democratic states. Citizenship is about inclusion and exclusion, and that's why one of the areas of great work has always been about citizenship and difference, be they ethnic difference, racial difference, gender. Feminists have demonstrated that according to traditional political theory, the citizen is actually a male, and white. But the issue is whether you cast aside the language of citizenship, whether you try to reinvent it, or whether you try and draw upon elements of the language that can be more inclusive.

IAN: As you talk about it you start off by saying that citizenship is by definition membership of a political community – the state – so therefore the language of citizenship is about governance. But you then move on to talk about it in a much more ethical universalist kind of way which goes beyond the limits of the nation-state. It implies being citizens of the world. It's a notion of being participants in a conversation – which is what I like – but that suggests that you can actually disconnect it from formal membership of a nation-state.

PATRICIA: But it can be a language of resistance to current forms of governance . . . when we talk about citizenship we are actually talking about the kind of society we want to create . . . When we develop a more inclusive notion of citizenship – one based on our equal status as human beings – that is actually saying that is the kind of society we want to have. An entrepreneurial notion of citizenship says that we want a competitive society.

JANICE: Anna Yeatman – at a conference in Brisbane in 1996 – quoted Hannah Arendt, who talked about human beings as 'sitting around a table' and necessarily having to live together . . . Yeatman, who was talking principally about difference, said that the task of citizenship . . . is to learn to live with those who are incommensurably different. So, it's about moving beyond membership of this imagined political community . . . [which] may require that you belong to a particular cultural or ethnic community. I think the language of citizenship is useful because it talks about human beings as moral or ethical equals – ethical entities in their own right – whereas the econometric language of the citizen as consumer doesn't. So, there are . . . ways in which people are trying to rescue, or revive, or recover some of the positive elements of citizenship.

IAN: It seems to me what you and Patricia have been saying is that intrinsic to the notion of citizens is a conception of governance. It's how we articulate our membership of a kind of community and how we should be ruled. So it can't just be a language of resistance and opposition.

Citizenship, status and belonging

JANICE: Citizenship is a formal status. In political terms it is citizenship which entitles people to participate in decision making; i.e. to vote. That's the bare minimum . . . [but citizenship] is also an imagined community . . . As a citizen you have a right to participate in decisions that affect you. That's part of the sort of society that Patricia is talking about . . . That political status is the necessary but not sufficient condition [for] those other more social elements of citizenship that we have been concerned with since at least the beginnings of this century, for example Marshall's notion of social citizenship as necessary for people to be able to participate more equally.

PATRICIA: What's the status of children?

JANICE: They are not formal citizens – they're potential or proto-citizens – which is one of the reasons why citizenship or civic education is always important. To be a citizen you are supposed to be a rational individual and children aren't considered to be rational individuals ... One of the things that education does is train children in the forms of rationality which equip them to act as rational equals – adults – i.e. as citizens.

ALAN: I've got a bit of a problem with some of the direction of the argument which I think you are reciting. You mentioned some ideas of community. If you look at some of the arguments ... of the American feminist philosophers such as Iris Marion Young, the attention has shifted to the exclusionary implications of notions of community. When one makes appeal to citizenship – or some notion of the circumscribed community – there's always going to be some group that's not included. It has become apparent with AIDS where assumptions are made about sexual communities which don't relate to the ways in which people conduct themselves. For example, there are [assumed to be] discrete homosexual citizens and discrete heterosexual citizens. That's why some of the safe-sex campaigns have been misguided. The infection has been spread by avowedly heterosexual men having sex with other men. So the limits of the modernist discourse about having fixed identities ... have become apparent ...

PATRICIA: It occurs to me that if one tries to imagine what you would have if you didn't have the language of citizenship, you would have the language of the market ... What the language of the market produces ... is winners and losers...putting people in exchange relationships. You have competitors, bargainers and contractors. In contrast, the social-democratic language tends to produce insiders and outsiders on a quasi-moral basis. There is no getting away from the fact that the language of citizenship will always produce an in group and an out group. There's something about the very language which is suspect.

IAN: Yes, but your point relates to the rhetoric of community, that's what's suspect. The alternative language is that of civil society – where you create a space where people can form associations, talk to each other, disagree with each other with varying degrees of belonging. So the language of community is all right in certain ways. But it can't be pushed too far ...

JANICE: So we are saying we like the idea of a loose sort of community but not a tightly integrated community in which the criteria of membership are too restrictive?

Practical concerns

ALAN: How does the new environmental discourse fit into this? I'm thinking about the public health discussions about responsibility to other species, future generations . . . and other family members; i.e. through genetic health . . . and claims about one's consumption. There seems to be an increasing emphasis on duties as well as rights relating to membership in an international community. Some of that could be seen as challenging some of the older orthodoxies about conceptions of citizenship. But also about incorporating people in new ways – creating a whole series of other responsibilities – which constrain individuals.

JANICE: Well there certainly is a whole field of environmental or green democratic theory. And there are discussions of what's called ecological citizenship which does see all human beings on the planet together and therefore having a form of membership of a community. That community, incorporated in the notion of ecological citizenship, includes future generations . . . and non-human species. It is [an] almost transcendental notion of citizenship which is broadening the community to which the citizen belongs – beyond the nation-state and beyond the existing generation and beyond the human species.

IAN: Can I come back to the issue of ecological citizenship? For example, our local council asks us to do the right thing and recycle our rubbish. So there are a whole set of disciplines that we adopt. And governments have employed a whole series of programmes which train us, making use of the language of citizenship. You have corporations that become good corporate citizens, using more energy-efficient technologies and so on. It seems to me that's a bit like the neo-liberal concept of citizenship we have been critiquing, because it is a top-down thing. On the other hand, you have activists who are saying – in a language of citizenship – we should be caring about the future of the planet. The notions are similar, but the positions from which they are articulated give them quite different meanings.

ALAN: I think some of the ecological arguments are ones which on the face seem quite clear, like 'act locally, think globally', but when you put them into practice, the contradictions soon become apparent – one example is Fremantle [in Western Australia] where we have tried to engage people in recycling with fortnightly [rubbish] pick-ups. Immediately there was a reaction from sections of the community whose lifestyles and values had been offended by it. An assumed notion of the common good and a notion of responsible citizenship was at work there . . .

IAN: So what's the implication: that those who protested against it were benighted and ecologically irresponsible? When you have councils and state governments saying: let's introduce this re-cycling programme, there is pressure for everyone to become more ecologically responsible. At one level it's fine, it's a good thing to do, but I have a suspicion that while it is one way to get populations to become ecologically responsible it also deflects attention from other corporate practices which are much more systemically destructive. When you have local powerless greenies saying we have to be more ecologically responsible it's a different discourse because it's a discourse of protest rather than a discourse of control.

JANICE: Ian's earlier comment about citizenship being negotiated and open-ended is the sort of thing that Anna Yeatman is talking about and is the sort of thing some people see as what should be underlying or underpinning citizenship education in schools. In other words, pointing out to young proto-citizens . . . that the task of citizenship is . . . learning how to live with people who are different from ourselves. Now that's about negotiation. It doesn't present citizenship as a static concept into which you have to be . . . initiated. It says that citizenship is something that human beings construct through negotiation. It is socially con-structed through human negotiation, through human agency . . .

IAN [to Patricia]: What do you think about the danger of cooption: for example, the cooption of the feminist critique of patriarchy, say, in equal opportunity legislation and bureaucratic practices?

PATRICIA: For sure, though in the act of coopting . . . rationalities of governance are also changed. Equal opportunity is a case in point – it has been coopted – but the forms of governance have changed. Not as much as we would have wished, but I think the changes have been reasonably significant.

JANICE: And you also realise how useful those practices are – even though they are coopted – when you go somewhere those conditions do not apply.

ALAN: . . . Once the representational policies have been established, in terms of committees, etc., the next thing is to step back and ask questions about representational practices. I think that's happening now with feminism and other groups. People are saying . . . how representative are these people of the groups they are claiming to represent?

PATRICIA: Going to some other practical implications . . . say health. I think that an inclusive or social democratic citizenship discourse suggests that the only way in way in which claims can be rationed is in relation to the person's need for that service. So there's no way in which private insurance should influence access to services. There's no way in which private insurance should be directing services away from the public sector.

JANICE: You are talking about specific practices and I was thinking about . . . the notion of 'mutual obligation' which recently has been used in Australia to legitimise young unemployed people being required to work for their unemployment benefits. In fact, there is no *mutual* obligation; rather there is a one-way obligation of the young person to the community. Citizenship can challenge that one-way obligation and say that 'mutual obligation' means just that.

IAN: But I'd take it further because John Howard [the Prime Minister of Australia] used the notion of mutual obligation most recently to say to industry that they had an obligation to provide jobs. And, at one level, you would say that's great. But I reacted against that and I would do so on the grounds of citizenship because what is really [happening] is the opting out of government redistribution through taxation and welfare spending. It seems it establishes a kind of charity relationship rather than a justice relationship – that whether you like it or not we are a political community in which the state will act to redistribute.

JANICE: I think it's that which underlies the real sense of disquiet, even horror, that I have for the notion of private prisons, because it is, say, Prisons Incorporated engaging in punishment, or protection of the community – or whatever you see prisons for – rather than the community itself, as manifested in and by the government, or the state.

ALAN: Isn't there some notion of . . . duty of care; the notion that has evolved over a long period of time about caring for people's basic material welfare, and when that's left to the market there is no umpire to oversee that this condition is fulfilled?

PATRICIA: Well, there can be. With things like private prisons, the government can build in certain regulatory controls; for example, occupational health and safety standards apply across the private sector . . . But ultimately, you are right . . . The thing about Howard asking business to be involved . . . your objection certainly stands if this is simply a way of privatising the job. But if it is not simply that, if it is an attempt to actually create a society in which industry is seen as involved in the production of social capital as well as financial capital . . . then it seems better.

IAN: I agree. It's the connection between state and civil society. What you are arguing for is a flourishing civil society with lots of social capital. The notion of mutual obligation expresses this. But it does depend on having a state which is involved in fostering a civil society. My point is that the Howard government has been characterised by off-loading rather than facilitating.

Stakeholders and mutuality

JANICE: . . . The notion of a 'stakeholder society' that the Blair government is supposed to work around involves partnerships in a flourishing civil society. One would like to hope that is one way of moving towards what you're advocating, Ian.

PATRICIA: Do you think it is?

JANICE: I think it is the intent that underlies some of the language. Whether it will necessarily translate into practice is still to be determined. But it is an attempt to challenge the new right and neo-liberalism and say that social capital is important and all people are stakeholders in this society. It is an attempt to do so.

I don't want to sound too Pollyanna-ish, but having the language of a stakeholder society and community . . . is better than not having it. It may then be a resource to be drawn on. It can be used as an organising [principle] . . . like mutual obligation. Use that language to organise resistance . . .

PATRICIA: That's what the idea of a stakeholder society might be trying to do but I still don't like it . . . I'm still worried about it . . . I prefer the idea of a 'mutual society'. Mutuality doesn't imply sameness. What it does imply is a shared thing. So we can have a mutual risk which means we share the risk. And it implies reciprocity, because it recognises difference and interdependence. Stakeholder I don't like because it has very much a self-interest. Mutuality has both an element of self-interest . . . but there is also an element of not so much altruism, but a recognition of our common humanity.

JANICE: The insurance companies like National Mutual and AMP [Australian Mutual Provident Society] were mutual provident societies. They were about that interconnectedness. They didn't have stakeholders or shareholders, 'til they were demutualised, which is, after all, a form of privatisation. They came out of the days when there was no welfare state, when people joined together to protect each other from misfortune. Ironically, as we look to recover the sense of mutual, all of these institutions are being privatised!

ALAN: At the moment maybe you've got a resurgence of that: people forming their own banks in response to the big organisations which have got bigger and more remote from the people they are supposed to serve. For me, that's a very effective form of resistance . . .

PATRICIA: I think that the language of 'we-ness' shouldn't demand any more of people than a recognition of roughly our common human condition; that we share certain things like birth, death, despair, happiness – certain things that come with the job of living.

IAN: A universal human nature?

JANICE: No, a universal human experience – that we sit around the same table.

PATRICIA: However, mutuality can't stand on its own: it has to be accompanied by a commitment to redistribution and social justice.

Equality and redistribution

ALAN: We haven't talked a lot about that: the language of redistribution – the broader context, it's very constrained, it's a capitalist relationship . . . [we] need to think of what is actually counter discursive.

JANICE: When you say I'm a citizen, implicit in that is that I am an equal citizen. A formal equality is part of the language of citizenship . . . there is an ongoing tradition that contrasts material circumstances with the formal equality of citizenship. And that's a language of resistance to forms of governance that result in greater inequality and differential economic circumstances.

ALAN: I suppose we should raise questions about the term 'inequality' . . . Some of the injustices that arise are not adequately addressed in terms of a discussion about inequality – class, ethnicity, gender. Some of the imperatives of neo-liberal rule . . . create injustices which don't align with those inequalities. I'm thinking about something like being flexible and mobile in one's work, and the new employment practices around the new [Australian Federal Government] agency, Centrelink. If the jobs are available one should go where the jobs are, regardless of the implications. This might lead to regional disparities, or disturbances in the family, which may cut across these traditional divisions.

JANICE: That's what I was saying: the neo-liberal governance models and practices will tend both to maintain existing forms of inequality and also create new ones.

IAN: David Marquand in *The Unprincipled Society* asks the question of what explains the loss of support for the social democratic welfare state in the 1970s and 1980s. His argument was that the Beveridge welfare state enacted a system of redistribution without addressing the question of social ontology. The question of alternatives needs to go deeper than the issue of equality of distribution to notions of mutuality and relationality – what makes us 'we' and not just 'I'. On the one hand, we have a sense that 'I' language is atomising, it reduces you to being a consumer, a self that is constructed in all sorts of ways. The problem of defining a language of 'we-ness' that is not co-ercive and unequal is quite difficult. At the heart of it, how do we find a sense of connectedness such that we are able to be ourselves to be free, but connected? It's always been a problem.

Citizenship and human rights

PATRICIA: What work does the language of citizenship do that the language of human rights does not do?

IAN: Well, it goes back right back to where you started. It brings into focus being a member of a political community. So it's a language of politics . . . The language of human rights by itself can be too abstract.

PATRICIA: Can I then pose another question . . . My aunt is in a nursing home for elderly people. She is dying, she is on morphine at the moment. Is there any way that the language of citizenship is relevant to her, or would we just use the language of respect for persons? . . .

JANICE: . . . We have a person in a nursing home. If she is a public patient and she is in a nursing home, that is part of the public health sector, then in a sense she can claim that care as a citizen. That's a citizenship entitlement.

PATRICIA: But that's where I think citizenship may do too much work. That is also claimable by your proto-citizens. Social rights seem to belong to people . . . because of respect for persons, they are owed decent treatment on an equal basis because they are persons, not because they are citizens. But my aunt has a long tradition as a citizen of which we cannot divest her. I don't know, is citizenship relevant here?

IAN: My answer to that question is that the respect for persons and the idea of citizenship go together, because the regard for people as citizens is a political expression of respect for persons. That's the force of extending the rights of citizens as wide as possible, and why we feel the problem of national citizenship to be arbitrarily exclusionary. That maps back on to the respect for people as persons *per se*. But conversely, unless you articulate respect for persons in terms of citizenship, it remains abstract and apolitical.

PATRICIA: So you are suggesting that the language of citizenship is derived from the more general principle of respect for persons? If that is right, then the particular way which the language of citizenship has been hijacked by neo-liberalism . . . is fraught with problems in the fundamental sense that it has separated itself from respect for persons.

IAN: However, the converse is important for me, coming from a Christian tradition . . . Within the mainstream church system there is this formal regard for persons – each person is equal before God, but none the less politically it continues to be hierarchical. How do you connect this line of reflection with poststructuralism?

PATRICIA: Well, I think you probably can't. Poststructuralism does not deal with ethical or practical concerns, not in that sort of way. It doesn't rule them out but that's not what it's primarily about. It's not the task at hand.

ALAN: It does depend on the kind of poststructuralist you are, Patricia. We discussed in an earlier chapter that some post-structuralists stand at the more critical end and others at the more diagnostic, non-normative end. Some are clearer about asking normative questions and locating themselves in a norma-tive framework. So I guess I'd be wary of making general statements of that kind.

PATRICIA: That's true.

Connection and division

PATRICIA: If I walk out of that door and bang my head on the door jamb – you three are all going to go 'oohh'. Now that's not to do with shared values; as Janice said before, it's to do with a shared experience.

IAN: But the crucial thing is to extend that 'oohh' beyond you to people towards whom we have no cultural [or] ethnic affinity. A capacity to extend that fellow feeling is not a natural universal or given.

PATRICIA: Maybe it's not given. But there is a modest case for it: a characteristic which humans have to a greater or lesser extent to be concerned about other people.

IAN: My reading of Charles Taylor is that he was showing that our moral intuitions – such as a sense of universal human dignity – have a distinctive history which is shaped by a whole range of practices, such that they wouldn't be self-evident in the past.

PATRICIA: Yes, we can acknowledge that respect for persons is a recent invention. But what I'm going on about – in relation to shared experience – is the kind of principle that lies behind ecological thinking. It's what connects us . . . is as important as what separates us. There is an awful lot that connects us. Talking about other species, I'm always fascinated when I see the skel-eton of a tiny lizard in my garden. That lizard is so similar to us.

IAN: The simple point is that even that kind of recognition is discur-sively constructed. We now live in a time when the ecological orientation encourages that kind of awareness.

PATRICIA: It would also happen in Aboriginal culture!

IAN: Yes, but not in our European modernity . . . Yet if you go back to medieval times, and notions of a great chain of being, there was a different sense of connectedness. It's the enlightenment that brings that sense of separateness.

ALAN: Feminists often talk about embodied knowledge as the basis of mutuality – feminists like Liz Grosz – there is a whole range of different feminists. From what I've read, some of it is a bit essentialist; it's often based on biology. They talk about difference in and of itself. But for me, difference is usually with reference to its opposite. I'm just wondering where one can take the argument about an embodied mutuality.

PATRICIA: Yes, it has to be made more practical. Let's take health and say that we have a shared common mutual risk of illness. There is a very practical way that it makes sense to pool our resources so that everyone is supported within the public sector. That is the practical side of it. Also, it probably makes ethical sense in a profound way. The trouble with neo-liberalism is that it appeals to the self-interest more than the empathetic side.

IAN: Michael Ignatieff's *The Needs of Strangers* touches this at the level of how we extend that sense of connectedness beyond the local to global connection, which becomes important in relation to communicable diseases – strains of the flu, etc., in so far as they are linked to particular kinds of social conditions. It would be in our self-interest to contribute much much more to global health care because of that sense that we are all in it together. But, unfortunately, political action doesn't happen because we don't have that sense of obligation.

PATRICIA: To take a domestic example: I can cook a chicken for my dogs because I have a much closer sense of connection with my dogs than I do with the poor chicken. But that's something you have to live with. More distant or different species are less likely to attract that [empathy]. And this goes right back to the thing about citizenship and some of the uses of attaching it to a particular territory. It is useful to talk about being citizens of the world, but it is kind of big to do so.

IAN: But that's what globalisation is doing. Coca Cola culture inculcates a sense of connectedness.

JANICE: But it's connectedness mediated through consumer culture, whereas there's a whole cosmopolitan literature, ideas of cosmopolitan citizenship which are similarly global but not based in consumer culture.

PATRICIA: That advert of people from around the world drinking Coke certainly doesn't improve one's capacity to feel for people who are drinking polluted water and dying of it, because the images are of healthy people drinking Coke.

JANICE: Also it isn't pointed out that Coke might cost a month's salary!

IAN: However, even though it's very truncated, when the Coke ad says it's because you drink Coke that you are part of a universal family, it does reinforce the idea that you have something in common with people in Africa.

It seems a bit odd to come to the end of this book talking about the dubious universalism of Coca Cola ads. Yet in fact Coke is emblematic of the discursive challenge posed by a globalising neo-liberalism and reminds us of the ways in which the micro world of everyday practice is connected to increasingly global techno-economic processes. At the beginning of 1998, Murdoch University management distributed a new set of student ID/library cards. Featured on the back of these cards were the logos for Coca Cola and Smith's Crisps. At one level this was a neat revenue-raising initiative, consistent with the consumption patterns of many students and the accepted presence of Coke machines around the campus. Yet at another level it was emblematic of the redirection of university policy: to become a more entrepreneurial 'degree factory' competing in the global educational market place.

Poststructuralist analysis helps to make visible the discursive reforming of everyday practices. We are able to see the connections between seemingly trivial, necessary or rational reforms introduced for reasons of productivity, competition or greater consumer choice. We are therefore perhaps more mindful of what is being lost and better able to resist the smooth cooption of the language of civic life.

References

Ignatieff, M. (1984) *The Needs of Strangers*, London: Chatto and Windus.

Marquand, D. (1988) *The Unprincipled Society: New Demands and Old Politics*, London: Cape.

Yeatman, A. (1996) 'Democratic theory and the subject of citizenship', paper presented at the Culture and Citizenship Conference, Brisbane, Queensland, Australia, October.

Index